Hysterectomy

How to deal with the physical
and emotional aspects

Melbourne
OXFORD UNIVERSITY PRESS
Oxford Auckland New York

OXFORD UNIVERSITY PRESS

Oxford London Glasgow New York Toronto
Delhi Bombay Calcutta Madras Karachi
Kuala Lumpur Singapore Hong Kong Tokyo
Nairobi Dar es Salaam Cape Town
Melbourne Auckland
and associate companies in
Beirut Berlin Ibadan Mexico City Nicosia

National Library of Australia
Cataloguing-in-Publication data:
Dennerstein, Lorraine.
    Hysterectomy.

    Bibliography. ˙
    Includes index.

    ISBN 0 19 554371 8.
    ISBN 0 19 554366 1 (pbk.).

    I.   Hysterectomy. I. Wood, Carl, 1929-.
    II.   Burrows, Graham D. (Graham Dene).
    III. Title.
618.1'453

Typeset by Meredith Typesetters, Melbourne
Printed in Hong Kong
Published by Oxford University Press, 7 Bowen Crescent, Melbourne
OXFORD is a trademark of Oxford University Press

Contents

Acknowledgements   7

Introduction   9

1 Why Hysterectomy?   11

2 Anatomy and Action: Where, What and How?   19

3 Sexual Satisfaction   28

4 Disease and Disorder: What is Wrong   40

5 The Types of Hysterectomy and the Dangers   59

6 Emotions: Coping with your Feelings   72

7 Practicalities: Before, During and After Surgery   83

8 The Menopause   97

9 Hormone Therapy: Effects and Side Effects   107

10 Life is What You Make It   114

Further Reading   123

Glossary   124

Index   129

To the women who have helped us in our studies.

Acknowledgements

We gratefully acknowledge the help given by Mr Warren Shepherd who drew the illustrations; Mrs Gertrude Rubinstein who compiled the glossary and index, Miss Lois Preston for advice on pelvic exercises and Mrs Millie Gerrard who typed and retyped the manuscript.

Introduction

This book has been written to help you understand your body, evaluate your symptoms, make an informed decision about surgery, and have an accurate knowledge of the way in which having a hysterectomy will affect you. We believe that this information will help you to make a healthy adjustment to the operation.

Our concern that such information be available to women began in 1975 when we interviewed many women who had undergone hysterectomy. We were appalled to find that the sexual relationships of many of these women had worsened after the operation. Women who lost interest in sex usually had fears that they would be altered sexually or in femininity by the operation. These fears were based on a lack of knowledge or an incorrect knowledge of the operation. Often they were triggered by unhelpful remarks made by friends or relatives. It became self-fulfilling: negative expectations led to changes in sexual behaviour.

Our belief that correct and accurate knowledge would prevent such problems has recently been tested in Israel. Women who had undergone hysterectomy attended a group meeting before leaving hospital. They were given information about their bodies and the effects of the operation and were encouraged to ask questions. These women made a much better adjustment to the operation, having fewer sexual or emotional problems than did women in the same hospital unit who were not given the opportunity to attend the group session. In our own study very few women had discussed their anxieties about the operation with their doctor. Women often reported that after being informed that hysterectomy would be needed, they were 'stunned'. Subsequently, they were unable to recall any discussion.

This book is not intended to substitute for discussion with your doctor. Rather it is meant to supplement your discussions with both your doctor and your partner. It is hoped that while reading this book you will identify problems and questions you wish to discuss further with your doctor.

1 Why Hysterectomy?

Hysterectomy is an operation which involves considerable physical and psychological stress. So too do many other types of surgery. But there has been an alarming increase in the frequency of hysterectomy. Hysterectomy is the most common major operation performed on women in the US and Australia. In 1973, 690,000 hysterectomies were performed in the US and in 1975 more than 25 000 hysterectomies were performed in Australia. Using other information available in Australia, it has been calculated that at the rate of surgery performed in 1975, 42 per cent of women will have a hysterectomy by the age of sixty-five. This is a conservative estimate, and it is quite possible that half the women will eventually have a hysterectomy.

Why should so many operations of this type be done? Most people would expect hysterectomy to be carried out because of disease of the uterus or associated organs, such as the ovaries, or both. These diseases include fibromyomata, endometriosis, severe or recurrent pelvic infection, prolapse, and cancer and are described in Chapter 4. Does this mean that pelvic disease occurs in nearly half the US and Australian female population? The answer is no. Very often the uterus removed is normal. Why are so many women undergoing hysterectomy in the absence of any disease?

MENSTRUATION

Women may seek relief from menstrual pain or bleeding through surgery. Community surveys in Australia demonstrate a high incidence of menstrual complaints. It is possible that an increase in these complaints may be related to an increase in smoking and drinking alcohol because these habits are associated with menstrual complaints. It is also possible that women in the Western world may now perceive as abnormal, menstrual blood loss or discomfort or both which would previously have been tolerated. This lowered tolerance of menstruation may be the result of the long-term use of the oral contraceptive pill. The oral contraceptive pill usually produces a marked reduction in the amount of bleeding and discomfort a woman experiences. Women are often advised to stop the 'pill' after the age of thirty-five and use other forms of contraception. Some women then find the return to 'normal' menstruation intolerable.

When women complain of heavy periods it does not necessarily mean that they are having a heavy blood loss. Prolonged heavy blood loss would lead to anaemia and ill-health, and hysterectomy is justifiable to prevent this. When women who complain of heavy periods are studied, only 50 per cent show evidence of an increased blood loss, and only a much smaller percentage are anaemic. Blood may comprise only 20 per cent of the total fluid content of menstruation, but this component is very important in determining therapy. The number of sanitary pads or tampons used bears little or no relationship to the actual amount of blood lost. Other factors also influence the amount of blood lost. In many primitive societies, for example, menstrual flow is scanty and usually only lasts one day. Nutrition may be an important factor.

Regular menstruation is an artefact of modern society. In more primitive societies, the menarche or first period occurs later, the menopause earlier, and pregnancy and prolonged breast feeding (with associated lack of periods) occupies much of the interim period.

In an evolutionary sense we have not had time for our bodies to adjust to the tremendous changes wrought by modern contraceptive technology. This may be another major reason for women expressing dissatisfaction with their periods and seeking hysterectomy in Western countries.

There are now available medications which help reduce the amount of bleeding and pain. These may not be acceptable to all patients or completely successful in eradicating symptoms. Nevertheless they are worth trying before considering surgery. These medications are discussed further in Chapter 4.

A woman's emotional state may also influence the amount of menstrual blood loss and discomfort and the woman's tolerance of, and perception of it. Studies in the UK and US have found an extraordinarily high percentage of women (55 to 57 per cent) to be suffering from significant emotional illness before having hysterectomies. The incidence of such symptoms in the general population is only 12 to 14 per cent. The main types of psychiatric problems suffered were depression and anxiety.

What do these findings mean? It is possible that some of the women may have developed anxiety about the forthcoming operation. In the UK study, women had been waiting to have the operation for up to one year. When it is known that an operation is needed, such a long wait may produce increased anxiety. Interestingly, over half of the UK patients with psychiatric problems had significantly improved when interviewed eighteen months after the operation.

It is also possible that women with psychological problems or some inner distress go to doctors with gynaecological symptoms. In our society there are commonly held negative attitudes to mental illness. Women with psychological distress may tend to present to their doctor saying 'I feel sick' rather than 'I feel sad or miserable or nervous'. Our medical system seems to encourage this focus on physical complaints rather than on emotional ones. As one of our patients remarked after hysterectomy, 'I go to the doctor when I feel bad, but I always seem to get the wrong thing', by which she meant operations, instead of treatment of her emotional problems. When people feel depressed or anxious they often focus on bodily symptoms and tend to perceive these more negatively.

Disorders of the mind may also adversely influence the menstrual cycle. The menstrual cycle is controlled hormonally by hormones secreted from the brain. The secretion of these brain hormones may be influenced by emotions. It is possible that women wih signicant emotional problems will find their menstrual cycle adversely affected. When the psychological problems are treated, menstrual problems may also be alleviated. See Figure 1.

These implications are important for the woman about to undergo hysterectomy. She should try and assess whether her symptoms reflect any emotional distress or stressful situations in her life. If she thinks they do, she should discuss her feelings frankly with her family doctor.

GYNAECOLOGISTS

Gynaecologists have a major influence in the rate of hysterectomy because they must make the final recommendations that such an operation is necessary. Women need to be aware of the factors which influence the gynaecologist to choose surgery. In making a diagnosis the gynaecologist relies on the description of the illness provided by the patient and an examination of the patient. Sometimes further investigations are carried out, such as blood tests, hormone investigations, or curettage of the uterus. A diagnosis is then made. In making this diagnosis, doctors rely heavily on the woman's perception of symptoms. Yet, as already described, it may be

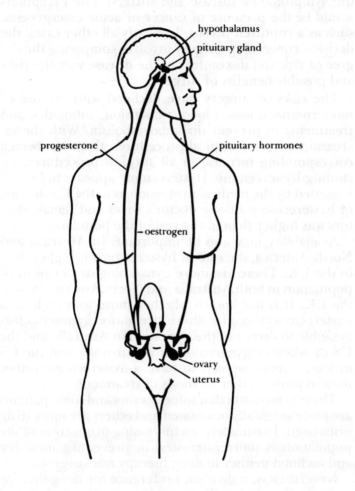

Figure 1 Hormone production

unrealistic to expect women to be accurate reporters of such symptoms as blood loss. Many of the reasons for surgery depend upon a woman's feelings in relation to the symptoms or disease she suffers. The exceptions would be the presence of cancer or acute emergencies, such as a ruptured uterus. In nearly all other cases, the decision concerning surgery involves comparing the degree of risk and discomfort of the disease with the risks and possible benefits of surgery.

The risks of surgery have declined with the use of modern anaesthesia, blood transfusion, antibiotics, and treatments to prevent thromboembolism. With the increasing safety of surgical procedures, there has been a corresponding increase in all surgical procedures, including hysterectomy. Hysterectomy appears to be well regarded by the medical profession as in the US the rate of hysterectomy among doctor's wives and female doctors was higher than in the rest of the population.

Availability may also be important. In Australia and North America, the rate of hysterectomy is higher than in the UK. There are more gynaecologists per head of population in both Australia and North America than in the UK. It is not known whether more women have a hysterectomy because there are more gynaecologists available to carry out the operation in Australia and the US or whether gynaecologists in Australia and the US influence more women to have a hysterectomy rather than to pursue other methods of treatment.

There is no doubt that some doctors and some patients are more surgically orientated and others are more drug orientated. Fortunately, an increasing proportion of the population is more interested in preventive medicine and inclined neither to drug therapy nor surgery.

Nevertheless, individual preference for drug therapy or surgery may significantly affect the final choice of treatment. Unfortunately, many gynaecologists have not been trained to recognize the hidden emotional problems in women who go to see them with gynaecological complaints. This is why it is particularly important for you to consider frankly whether emotional problems are present in your case and to discuss them with your doctor.

OTHER FACTORS

Fashion can influence the incidence of an operation. The frequency with which women relate experiences of hysterectomy in either a favourable or unfavourable light not only suggests its importance but also may create an expectancy among other women to have a hysterectomy. Anxiety may also contribute to the situation. An increase in media reports about cancer, pre-cancer, or other menstrual problems may increase women's anxiety about their health. Hysterectomy is an effective assurance in avoiding some of these problems, particularly cancer.

Some women have the operation as an alternative to sterilization, particularly if they wish to stop menstruation. But preventive hysterectomy is not popular in Australia, although it is practised in some countries. Preventive hysterectomy is based on the notion that after the uterus has served the purpose of childrearing it is a useless organ and a potential threat to good health. Most would not agree with this view because the uterus is important psychologically to many women. The reasons for removing the uterus as a preventive measure are to avoid uterine cancer, which affects 3 per cent of the female population, to put an end to menstrual problems, which affect 15 per cent of the population, to avoid the need for contraception, to avoid anxiety about pregnancy, cancer, and menstrual problems, and to give women the freedom to pursue occupations outside motherhood where menstruation is seen to be a disadvantage. The reasons against preventive hysterectomy are the risk of suffering physical complications as a result of the operation, the possibility of depression after surgery, and the pain, loss of time, and cost of having surgery. On balance, there is a very slight saving in terms of life from preventing cancer when the women who die from hysterectomy are also considered. It is possible that preventive hysterectomy may become more common, particularly in women who do not regard the uterus as important for their emotional well-being.

Many factors play a part in influencing the high rate of hysterectomy. When well selected this operation may significantly improve the quality of your life. The appropriate selection of this operation depends on you and your doctor. Your adjustment to the operation will be influenced by your beliefs and your expectations of the operation. The following chapters will provide you with a sound knowledge to help you to make the decision about surgery and to adapt to the operation successfully.

2 Anatomy and Action: Where, What and How?

WHERE IS THE UTERUS?

Most people have difficulty identifying where an organ is in the body. The heart is commonly recognized as a muscular pump lying in the chest, and its position can be imagined easily because the beat of the heart can be felt. The brain can also be located because it is confined by the bony skull behind the face. The uterus is more dif-

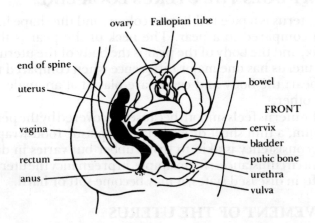

Figure 2: Cross-section of the body showing the position of the pelvic organs

ficult to localize because, although it is known to lie in the pelvis, it does not pulsate or lie close to bony surfaces.

If the pelvis is imagined as a box with the front side much shorter than the back, then the uterus lies centrally within this box. Some women are able to accurately locate the position of the uterus from contractions occurring during menstruation or during orgasm. But many women do not feel contractions and in others the pain of contractions is felt diffusely in the pelvis, or referred elsewhere to the abdomen or upper thighs.

The uterus has four neighbours: the vagina below, the bladder in front, the loops of bowel above, and the rectum or back passage behind (see Fig. 2). These neighbours are important as any enlargement or disease of the uterus may upset their function and lead to problems associated with the vagina (pain with sexual intercourse), the bladder (urination or micturition) or bowel (defaecation).

WHAT DOES THE UTERUS LOOK LIKE?

The uterus is a pale red-brown colour, and the shape has been compared to a pear. The neck of the pear is the cervix, and the body of the pear is the body of the uterus. The uterus has one major difference when compared to the pear: the body and cervix are placed at an angle to each other.

The uterus feels smooth because it is covered by the peritoneum, a thin sheet of material like plastic food wraps. The consistency is akin to firm rubber but varies in different circumstances; for example, in pregnancy the uterus is soft; in diseased states, it may become soft or hard.

MOVEMENT OF THE UTERUS

The uterus moves. It is able to move because it is placed in the centre of the pelvis by ligaments which run from the uterus to the neighbouring organs and bones (see Fig. 2). These ligaments are partly elastic tissue and partly muscle, and the uterus moves by give in the elastic part of the ligament or by active contraction of the muscle part of the ligament. The uterus changes its position according to posture and also according to activity of the neighbouring organs. When a woman stands, the uterus normally drops 1 or 2 centimetres, even when it is healthy. Dropping of the uterus is exaggerated in women who have weakened ligaments: the condition called 'prolapse'.

The uterus also may alter position in a forwards and backwards manner so that when you are lying on your stomach the uterus is closer to the front of the pelvis. When you are lying on your back, the uterus lies closer to the back of your pelvis. The change in position of the uterus with postural change may cause discomfort for some women during intercourse. The uterus also rotates. The fixed point in rotation is the junction between the body and cervix. The body of the uterus may be rotated forwards, called 'anteversion', or rotated backwards, called 'retroversion' (see Fig. 3). Most often the uterus stays in one position, either anteversion or retroversion. In some women, however, the uterus may rotate or flip itself from anteversion to retroversion or vice versa. Discomfort may occur if rotation takes place during coitus, or during examination by a doctor who is determining if the uterus can be moved.

The position of the uterus may also be influenced by

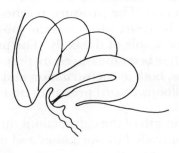

Figure 3 Possible positions of the uterus

what is happening to neighbouring organs. When the bladder is full, the uterus moves backwards and may rotate itself from anteversion towards retroversion. If the rectum is very full with faeces, the uterus may be pushed forwards. During intercourse, the penis pushes the uterus upwards. When diseases occur in the neighbouring organs, the uterus may also be displaced. Any lump or growth in a surrounding organ would displace the uterus and this can be in an upward direction if the growth is in the vagina, forwards if the growth is in the bowel, or backwards if the growth is in the bladder. Such displacement of the uterus is usually not recognized by the woman concerned, but on occasion there may be pain. Displacement of the uterus will affect the way the surgeon removes the uterus or neighbouring growths.

UTERINE MUSCLE AND CONTRACTIONS

Half the uterus consists of muscle. The muscle is different from that in the arms or legs because a woman cannot control when or how the muscle will contract.

The muscle has two main functions, to expel menstruation and to expel the fetus and placenta. During each month, the contractions of the muscle vary markedly. The uterus is least active when the embryo embeds in the lining of the uterus, nine to twelve days before the menses start. The muscle is most active at the time of menstruation and during labour. These contractions are very powerful. The pressure reached is only one-third less than the heart which has the job of pumping blood around the whole of the body. The pressure of the contractions has been measured by putting tiny balloons in the uterus, both at menstruation and during childbirth. These balloons record pressures up to 80 millimetres of mercury.

The strength of the contractions during the menstrual cycle is controlled by hormones and the nervous system. The hormones oestrogen and progesterone are secreted during the cycle and are responsible for the reduction in muscle activity at mid cycle. The strong contractions at menstruation are the result of two factors: the withdrawal of the hormones oestrogen and progesterone, and the release of powerful muscle stimulating substances called prostaglandins.

If one of the prostaglandins is produced in an excessive amount, the contractions at menstruation become too powerful and this results in pain. Drugs can now be given to reduce the production of prostaglandins in women with menstrual pain. These drugs act by stopping the production of prostaglandins or the action of prostaglandin on the muscle, thereby reducing contractions and also the pain.

The powerful contractions that some women notice during orgasm may be related to sexual stimulation of the nervous system with the release of hormones which contract the muscle or to the release of prostaglandins from the uterus as a result of stretching of the vagina and uterus by the penis.

Before puberty and after menopause, the uterus does not contract powerfully because the muscle is no longer under the strong influence of hormones.

The muscle of the uterus is neatly arranged in two different patterns. The outer muscle runs as a straight band from the cervix upwards over the back of the uterus then over the top and down the front wall back to the cervix. When this band of muscle contracts, it has a squeezing action so that any menses or blood in the cavity of the uterus can be easily expelled. The muscle under this long band is arranged differently. Bundles of muscle criss-cross over each other and surround blood vessels, which they can close by squeezing. This squeezing action over the blood vessels will help to control bleeding from the uterus at the time of menstruation or after birth.

NERVES SUPPLYING THE UTERUS

The nerves passing to and from the uterus are to some extent a mystery. There is a rich nerve supply, particularly to the cervix, and the nerves travel to blood vessels and muscle cells. Messages pass from the brain along the nerves and thereby can change the blood flowing to the uterus and also the amount of muscle contracting. The uterus, however, can function without the nerves. When the nerves are cut in experiments in animals, the uterus still functions during menstruation or labour. Cutting the nerves in the human reduces the pain perceived at menstruation because the nerve fibres carrying pain messages are cut. For a short time after the nerves are cut the periods may be heavier. Thus the nerves may affect the amount of blood lost during menstruation.

THE INNER LINING OF THE UTERUS OR ENDOMETRIUM

The uterus has an inner lining, called the 'endometrium', which changes each month. The endometrium is shed at the time of menstruation but grows again until either pregnancy or menstruation occurs. The growth of the endometrium is in two phases. In the first two weeks after the periods, the endometrium thickens and small circular rings (glands) develop in the endometrium. In the second half of the cycle, the thickening continues but to a lesser extent. The glands become filled with a fluid substance called 'secretion'. The secretion in the endometrium is important should pregnancy occur because the embryo has to burrow into the endometrium and sustain itself from nutrients in the secretion. If pregnancy occurs, a hormonal message is sent from the embryo to the mother enabling the ovaries to continue functioning so that the endometrium is sustained into pregnancy. If pregnancy does not occur, the ovary stops producing its hormones, and as a result the endometrium dies and is shed at the time of menstruation. Menstruation results from the failure of pregnancy to occur.

MENSTRUATION

Menstruation is a complicated process involving four important events: a change in hormone levels, death of the endometrium, the expulsion of the dead endometrium with blood, and the cessation of bleeding (see Fig. 4).

The hormone changes are mainly related to the cessation of production of oestrogen and progesterone by the ovaries and increasing production of prostaglandins by the uterus. As a result of the hormone changes, the blood vessels going to the endometrium close and this leads to the death of the endometrium and subsequent shedding of the endometrium into the uterine cavity. The vessels are also shed and so bleeding occurs.

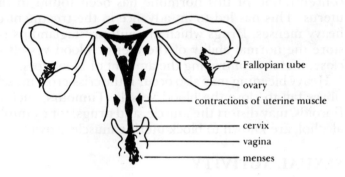

Figure 4 How menstruation occurs

The blood and endometrium are expelled into the vagina by powerful uterine contractions.

The cessation of bleeding is dependent upon three major factors: the constricting effect of the criss-cross muscle fibres on the blood vessels leading to the endometrium; the system of blood clotting which normally exists in the body; and the growth of new endometrium which re-lines the uterine surface. As bleeding from the uterus is dependent on so many factors, it is understandable that less is known about uterine bleeding than bleeding problems elsewhere in the body.

When any of the three major controlling systems are at fault, menstruation may be excessive; for example, women with bleeding disorders, where some of the clotting factors are deficient, suffer heavy menses. In addition, when the hormone production from the ovary is disturbed, common soon after puberty or immediately before the menopause, re-growth of the endometrium is affected and menstrual bleeding may be heavy. In these hormonal disorders, progesterone is not produced or the amount of oestrogen may be too little or too much.

High levels of the hormone, prostaglandin, have been found to cause heavy bleeding by opening blood vessels. In a number of women with heavy menses, increased concentration of this hormone has been found in the uterus. This has led to an advance in the treatment of heavy menses. Drugs which are anti-prostaglandins restore the normal ability of the uterine blood vessels to close, thereby controlling the amount of blood loss.

Heavy bleeding may also occur if the criss-cross muscle fibres fail to close the blood vessels. Tumours, such as fibroids, may distort the muscle, and drugs, for example, alcohol, are known to block uterine muscle activity.

SEXUAL ACTIVITY

When a woman becomes excited, the ligaments of the uterus contract and move the uterus upwards out of the pelvis. This is beneficial as the penis can move more freely in the lower part of the pelvis. The external opening of the cervix into the vagina is also wider during sexual activity and this may favour the passage of sperm into the uterus. During orgasm the uterus contracts and this may help the passage of sperm through the genital tract. It was thought that the uterus acted like a vacuum with a negative pressure inside it, sucking the sperm from the vagina. This does not occur, but the contractions may cause a favourable flow of fluid upwards in the tract or in some other way may stimulate the transport of sperm. Some women feel and enjoy uterine contractions that occur with orgasm.

THE MIND AND THE UTERUS

Women often wonder whether the mind controls the uterus. Although there is no obvious conscious control of the uterus by the mind, the mind influences the uterus in a number of ways. The psychological state can influence the hormone levels produced by the ovary through the intermediary action of the pituitary gland placed at the base of the brain. Changes in the production of hormones by the ovary will alter the endometrium and the muscle of the uterus. This in turn may affect menstruation by changing either the severity of contractions or the amount of blood loss.

In acute emotional states, the mind sends different messages along the nerves including those running to the uterus and these nerves are connected both to the muscle and blood vessels. Chemicals coming from the nerves cause contractions so that menstruation may be more painful. Furthermore, emotions may change the production of hormones released from other glands in the body (the adrenal, pituitary) and these can pass through the blood stream to the uterus where they may influence menstruation (see Fig. 1).

The uterus and brain are part of the one body. A malfunction (emotional or physical) of the brain may affect the uterus, or alternatively malfunction of the uterus, by causing pain or excessive bleeding, may affect the brain. It is also possible that some psychological states will not affect the uterus. It is clear from studies of women with menstrual disturbances that menstrual pain, in particular, may be related to psychological well-being. On the other hand the length of the period mainly depends on physical factors.

3 Sexual Satisfaction

Over the last few decades tremendous changes have taken place in attitudes to sexuality in most Western countries. Although earlier this century women tended to regard sex as a marital duty, today's women expect their sexual relationships to bring physical and emotional fulfilment. Unfortunately, most women today were raised with a legacy of negative attitudes to sex. Consequently, although their expectations have changed, there is still much sexual dissatisfaction. As lack or incorrect knowledge of sex are potent causes of sexual problems, it is important to consider what comprises sexual behaviour.

SEXUAL BEHAVIOUR

Sexual Desire

Sexual desire is an appetite or drive, one of the basic instinctual drives or needs which are present at birth and without which we could not as a species have survived. Other basic drives or needs include hunger, thirst, and aggression. One explanation for the sexual drive is that it is part of an instinct or need to reproduce. But lower animals cannot possibly know that mating results in reproduction. A simpler and more likely explanation is that fundamentally we engage in sex because it is pleasurable. That the sexual drive is present from birth may be observed in the obvious interest and pleasure of babies in cuddling and skin contact. The sexual drive is increased at puberty with the development of the genital organs and the production of sex hormones.

Sexual Response

The sexual drive leads to seeking some form of stimulation (physical, psychological or both) which produces a feeling of sexual excitement. During this excitement or arousal phase blood flow is increased, especially in the genital area of the body. Increased blood flow leads in the male to erection of the penis and in the female to the production of vaginal lubrication. With increasing arousal there is a build up of muscular tension until, at a peak level of excitement, the orgasm or climax occurs. Physically, the orgasm is caused by involuntary muscular contractions. In the male these contractions produce ejaculation. Vaginal contractions occur in the female but not all women are aware of them. Most women are aware of an intensely pleasurable experience, a peak of sexual excitement, followed by profound relaxation throughout the body.

The rapidity and degree of sexual arousal depends on many factors. These include the individual's own sexual desire and mood (anxiety and guilt can inhibit arousal), whether the environment is conducive or inhibitory, and the feelings towards the partner.

Sexual Activity

There is a wide variation between individuals in both the amount and type of preferred sexual activity. Some people derive sexual satisfaction from a single type of activity; others prefer many different techniques.

Satisfaction of the sexual drive may be achieved in different ways. For example, some gratification may occur using psychological means such as the use of fantasy. Sexual day-dreams form a frequent part of both men and women's thoughts. Sexual dreams also occur during sleep (wet dreams or nocturnal orgasms). Thoughts and fantasies are often combined with physical actions to enhance sexual pleasure. An important physical releasor of sexual tension is self-stimulation or masturbation. Almost all men and most women masturbate at some stage during their lives. Masturbation is not confined to adolescence but continues throughout life, whether or not there is a sexual partner. Previously it was thought that masturbation might be harmful and the cause of diseases varying from insanity to blindness. We now know that there are no harmful effects of masturbation and there may be many positive effects. By self-stimulation a person learns a great deal about his or her own sexual response, how to achieve sexual release, and what sexual satisfaction feels like. A common myth is that women who masturbate may become unable to enjoy sexual intercourse. But the reverse holds true. The woman who masturbates before marriage is more likely to achieve orgasm or full sexual satisfaction with her husband.

Petting or foreplay is an intensely pleasurable aspect of love-making. Many women attain full sexual release during foreplay, especially foreplay that involves direct rhythmic stimulation of the vulva. It is now known that some women are only able to achieve orgasm with such direct stimulation and this is thought to be perfectly normal. Direct stimulation may be provided by the partner's fingers or tongue (oral sex).

Intercourse or coitus is the major source of sexual release for men and is an important source of sexual pleasure for women. Some women reach orgasm during intercourse; others enjoy the feelings of intimacy, 'completeness', of being as close to each other as is possible.

Although sexual activity would be expected to occur as a response to sexual drive, there are other reasons. These include the desire to have a child, please one's partner, prove one's femininity, provide evidence of attractiveness, and to express affection or love.

COMMUNICATION

It is important to emphasize the uniqueness of each individual in the experience and expression of sexuality. Each of us has a different genetic make-up and is exposed to differing parental, social, cultural and religious influences. Individual experiences in relation to the sexual organs also add to our uniqueness. There is, consequently, a large range of sexual behaviour that is considered 'normal'. An implication is that no man or woman can automatically know his or her partner's preferences for sexual stimulation. A 'good' lover is the person who is able to elicit what his or her partner's sexual needs are. Communication, verbal and non-verbal, is thus vital to sexual enjoyment.

EFFECTS OF AGEING

Many myths surround sexuality in middle and old age. These include:
- no one over fifty ever makes love
- sexual activity should cease at the menopause
- interest in sex is abnormal for old people
- slower erection in the male is a sign that it will all be over soon.

These commonly held myths suggest negative attitudes by the community to the effects of ageing on sexuality.

What are the actual physical effects of ageing?

Females

With increasing age, arousal takes longer. Vaginal lubrication is slower to occur, and more direct and prolonged stimulation of the genitalia is often needed. The clitoral area is more easily irritated by direct stimulation, which is more effective if applied to adjacent areas. The orgasmic phase may become shorter and less intense. In women who have low levels of oestrogen following ovarian removal or ovarian failure at the menopause, thinning of the vulval, vaginal, and urethal tissues may occur with resultant pain during foreplay and intercourse. Some women develop painful uterine spasms during orgasm. This condition will not be a problem for the woman who undergoes hysterectomy.

Males

Arousal also takes longer for males so that erection of the penis occurs more slowly. The male who could become aroused merely on looking at his partner when younger now needs greater direct stimulation to the genitalia. With ageing, the time interval before ejaculation increases. The need and ability to ejaculate at each sexual contact are markedly reduced so that the male may reach a climax without ejaculating.

Following sex there is an increasing time before the male can be re-aroused. This time (the refractory period) varies greatly between individuals at any age. Thus slower erection in the male is not a sign of imminent impotence but rather an indication for more prolonged and pleasurable love-making.

Sexual Interest

There is a gradual decrease in sexual interest and activity with age. At the age of seventy-five, however, from one-quarter to one-half of all couples still have regular sexual intercourse. Neither men nor women lose their sexual needs or function with age. With good health and an interesting and interested partner, sex may last as long as life.

One study found that intercourse usually stops because of the male's inability to perform sexually rather than the woman's refusal.

ADVANTAGES OF AGEING

There are definite physical effects of ageing on sexuality. These changes are not necessarily disadvantageous. A major advantage of the need for prolonged arousal is that a couple now has the time for very enjoyable love-making. Women are now free to enjoy sex without fear of pregnancy and men are freed of the necessity to achieve full, quick erection and ejaculation. Prolonged sex play can give both partners pleasure and release from loneliness and tension. Sex may actually be therapeutic. Intercourse, for example, increases the adrenal gland output of hormones.

The potential for sexual pleasure begins at birth and ends at death. With the departure of children from the home, many couples reach an increased intimacy in their relationship and enjoy and value the privacy of being alone together again. With increased emotional maturity, the quality of the sexual interaction may change to a deeper form of human interaction and communication than was possible earlier.

REASONS FOR SEXUAL DISSATISFACTION

There are many causes of sexual problems. The most frequent cause is that the couple have general difficulties in their relationship. It is difficult to make love when you are making war. Hostility, anger, and resentment make poor bed-mates. Physical illness represents an increasing cause of sexual problems with age, either because of general ill-health or because of specific effects on the genitalia. Chronic inflammation of the tubes and ovaries, for example, may produce discomfort and pain during intercourse. Under these circumstances sexual interest would be expected to decrease. Alcohol and drugs may impair sexual response, especially the drugs used to treat high blood pressure. Chronic anxiety or depression also decreases both interest and arousal.

Some people with sexual problems show a pattern of behaviour which often includes anxiety during sexual arousal, avoidance of the sexual interaction, and no enjoyment of sex. With increased anxiety, the male may have difficulty getting an erection or may ejaculate prematurely, and the female's arousal is inhibited. The causes of this pattern of behaviour may be recent traumatic experiences or date back to early experiences in childhood where sexuality was either not discussed at all or portrayed negatively. Restrictions to sexual development include lack of knowledge, taboos applied by parents and religions, and specific traumatic experiences such as assault and rape. Painful intercourse caused by pelvic disease may be expected to lead to a pattern of sexual avoidance and disinterest.

Other sexual problems reflect particular conflicts of a person with his or her sexuality. These conflicts may reflect fears of losing control, of difficulty in forming close intimate relationships, of childbearing or rearing, and sometimes of homosexuality.

WHAT CAN BE DONE TO ENHANCE SEXUAL SATISFACTION?

If there have been sexual problems present for some time, most couples benefit from discussing them with a doctor or clinical psychologist who has been trained to deal with them. The therapy prescribed will vary depending on the cause.

The following principles may help to enhance your sexual enjoyment:

Increased Knowledge of Sexuality

It is never too late to learn to understand your physical and emotional behaviour. There are many books which you can use to increase your knowledge. Some of these are listed at the end of this book. Your partner should also read any books you select and you should both discuss their contents. Many doctors now have access to films or videotapes which visually portray normal sexual behaviour. Increased knowledge of sexuality should include an awareness of the changes to be expected with ageing so that these can be used to enhance your enjoyment.

Self-acceptance

This is an important concept for women. It is obviously difficult to share a part of your body of which you do not have a clear image. In the same way that you know clearly what your hand looks like even with your eyes closed, it is important to know what your vulva and vagina look and feel like. Most women find out by exploration during adolescence. Some women feel reluctant to look at the vulva unless they have an excuse (e.g. a lump, or rash, or episiotomy stitches). We have found that many women with sexual problems have not become comfortable about this area of their body, regarding it as dirty or messy or shameful. Sometimes women will say 'why should I change now? I was able to enjoy sex earlier in my marriage despite knowing little about that area'. Sometimes negative views can be overcome during the intense or infatuation phase of a relationship. As the relationship with the partner changes, however, your long standing

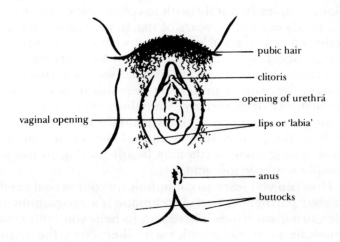

Figure 5 The vulva

attitudes to your body and to sexuality become more important.

How can you become more comfortable about your sexuality? The best way to overcome these negative attitudes to this important area of the body is to 'get in touch'. As part of your daily routine, for example, after showering, look at your vulva with a hand mirror and try and identify the parts shown in Fig. 5. You will probably feel uncomfortable at first, but if you continue daily you will overcome these feelings. The next step is to insert one finger into the vagina and explore it. The vagina is as long as your index finger and feels like a soft tube. It is elastic tissue so cannot be too big or small. It is also one of the cleanest parts of your body, having far fewer micro-organisms than are present, for example, in your mouth.

By accepting yourself, you will find it far easier to enjoy sharing this area of your body with your partner.

Communication of Sexual Needs

Many couples find it difficult to communicate their sexual needs even after years of marriage. Sometimes this reflects a lack of knowledge about what those needs are; this is especially true for the woman who has not masturbated. Others are aware of what sort of sexual stimulation they would prefer but fear this indicates some abnormality or perversity. Sometimes there is a lack of communication because the woman (or man) genuinely believes the partner should know. Others fear that verbally stating their needs may be off-putting to the atmosphere of the moment.

How can you learn to communicate your sexual needs to your partner? A useful technique is a programme of pleasuring exercises. These aim to help you both communicate more easily with each other, enjoy the giving and receiving of pleasure, and learn more of each other's sexual response. During these exercises it is suggested that you desist from intercourse so that more attention is given to the rest of the body as a sensual organ and the demand of intercourse is removed.

The exercises usually begin by each member of the couple taking it in turns to give the partner a general body massage. During this process the partner must tell the masseur his or her feelings and desires. Handcream may be used to facilitate the massage. During the first few sessions the massage should not extend to the genital area. After communication has been successfully developed during non-genital pleasuring, the massage can also extend to the breasts and genital area so that you each learn how your partner likes to be stimulated and caressed. At all times these exercises should be fun and not hard work! After genital pleasuring has been successfully achieved, the couple may proceed to intercourse.

These exercises are very well suited to couples in middle age because foreplay now becomes an important and necessary part of arousal if it has not been so until now.

Variety

Excitement is an important component of sexual arousal. One of the problems present in long-term relationships such as marriage is that the sexual relationship with time may become routine. One woman described her sexual interaction with her husband as 'a bore; we have had it the same way, in the same place, at the same time for the last twenty years. It is the last thing I do at night after cleaning my teeth'. Excitement and fun may follow variation of timing, setting, and technique. Ideas may be obtained from many sources, including some from the recommended reading in this book.

Frequency of Sex

Masters and Johnson have demonstrated that women who have intercourse at least once or twice a week are protected from some of the detrimental changes of hormonal depletion. With regular intercourse, the vagina continues to lubricate sufficiently during sexual arousal and does not constrict significantly in size. There is thus tremendous physical and psychological benefit to be obtained from regular and frequent sex. It appears that both the female and male sexual apparatus needs exercise to maintain functioning. With ageing, many people find it can be difficult to start again if sex has stopped for a time. This applies particularly to males. It is important never to drop sex for a long time: if you have no partner for the time being, keep yourself going alone with self-stimulation.

Hormones

Following ovarian failure, detrimental effects of thinning of the vagina, and vulval and urethal tissues may occur with consequent irritation during intercourse and proneness to infection. Vaginal lubrication may be delayed. Sexual desire or interest may also wane. Oestrogen therapy is known to alleviate all these changes. The oestrogen may be given locally as a cream or by tablets, injections, or long-lasting implant. The advantages and disadvantages of oestrogen must be evaluated for each individual. These are considered more fully in Chapter 9.

SEXUAL SATISFACTION AND HYSTERECTOMY

Hysterectomy is a major operation. Following the operation many women experience a drop in sexual interest for one to two months while they recover physically and emotionally from the stress of the operation.

When should you resume sexual relationships with your partner? You may have intercourse once the vagina has healed. Usually this has occurred by the time of the six-week post-operative check-up. Your doctor will advise you. If he or she does not comment after the examination ask about it.

Sometimes the first intercourse is a little uncomfortable, especially if you are anxious. Anxiety inhibits sexual arousal and the vaginal lubrication necessary for comfortable sex. The first intercourse is often made easier if your partner has been able to insert two fingers into the vagina comfortably during your love-making to prepare the way.

Although it may be six to eight weeks before intercourse is resumed, there is no need to waive general love-making. The demonstration of caring and enjoyment of each other is most beneficial both for your own recovery and for your relationship. The pleasuring techniques described above are most suitable for use at this time.

Although the operation of hysterectomy itself has no harmful physical effects on sexuality, fears about the operation may lead a woman and her partner to alter their sexual interaction, sometimes with disastrous results. For example, if the woman fears that she will be changed by the operation so that she becomes less attractive to her husband or less feminine, she will be very concerned about his approaches to her after the operation. Her husband may endeavour to be 'more understanding' following this major operation and make fewer sexual demands. She may then perceive this to mean that she is not attractive to her partner any longer. Some women will make persistent and continued demands on their partner to affirm to themselves that sexuality has not changed. Sexual demands may exceed the male's ability to respond, and he may find himself unable to 'perform', especially if this has been the first time during the marriage in which the woman has initiated sex. His reaction may be to avoid her. She may perceive this as another indication that she is not attractive sexually to her partner. Both members of the couple may then become depressed.

This is an unfortunate chain of events which is entirely preventable if the couple will communicate to each other their fears and feelings. Sex as an aspect of love-making will be more successful than sex undertaken as proof of femininity.

4 Disease and Disorder: What is Wrong

Malfunction of the uterus may cause a disturbance of menstruation, such as excessive or prolonged bleeding or pain. Less often pain or bleeding occurs at other times during the menstrual cycle.

Malfunction is caused by one of two basic mechanisms. In one, the uterus is damaged by disease, such as infection or cancer, and in the other, the uterus looks normal, but chemical changes cause the malfunction. It is important to understand the nature of the malfunction.

Basic information not only satisfies curiosity, but relieves anxiety about what is happening inside the body, facilitates communication between the patient and doctor, and helps determine both the seriousness of the problem and the choice of treatment: drugs, psychophysical therapy, or surgery.

MENSTRUAL PAIN

Menstrual pain is an important and common problem and is a symptom which may lead to hysterectomy.

Frequency

At least half of reproductive women suffer pain with menstruation, and in 15 to 30 per cent of women the pain occurs regularly each cycle. It is interesting that self-reporting of menstrual pain results in a higher incidence than when the frequency of menstrual pain is assessed by others, such as doctors. It is probable that many doctors do not consider the pain important unless it disrupts the woman's life.

Severity

In one in four women the pain is sufficiently severe to interfere with normal duties, either at work or home. The pain may last a few hours or a few days and is often associated with other symptoms such as headache, nausea, tiredness, and depression. It is not clear whether these symptoms result from the pain or are independent of the pain. The relationship between pain and other symptoms occurring at the time of menstruation is important. For example, you may wish to have a hysterectomy to gain relief from the pain and other symptoms such as headache and nausea. Relief from all symptoms may occur after hysterectomy. In some women, however, the associated symptoms of headache, nausea, and so on may persist after hysterectomy. It is important to try and unravel the relationship between the symptoms occurring at the time of menstruation in order to determine the possible benefits of hysterectomy.

Age

Menstrual pain is much more common in the young, the incidence being 80 per cent in the age group fifteen to nineteen years and 20 per cent in the age group forty to forty-nine years. This is important information because the normal expectation is for menstrual pain to decrease with age and should be taken into consideration before deciding on radical therapy, such as hysterectomy. If pain worsens with increasing age, it is very likely that some physical disease is present.

Childbirth

Another factor which is thought to relieve menstrual

pain is childbirth. Many women have been told that after a baby, the pain will disappear. This is not true. Pain is occasionally improved by childbirth, but in general the occurrence of pain in women with children is the same as in those without children.

Menstrual pain may be improved by contraceptive pill therapy. Nevertheless, one in four to five women still have menstrual pain despite contraceptive pill therapy. The modern contraceptive pill may be less effective because of the reduction in drug dosage. In making a choice between contraceptive pill therapy and hysterectomy, an alternative would be to use the outmoded higher dose pill. The risks of higher dose pills involve the serious problem of thromboembolism so that discussion with the doctor concerning alternatives is important. Some doctors have suggested that if menstrual pain is not relieved by the pill, psychological factors are responsible for the pain. This is not true. The psychological well-being of women who do not obtain relief with the pill is no different from those who do gain relief.

Social Habits

Menstrual pain is more common among smokers and drinkers. Alcohol is an effective muscle blocking agent and therefore may induce pain relief. Perhaps this has led women who suffer from pain to drink alcohol. Smoking may increase menstrual pain as nicotine in the cigarette increases muscle activity of the uterus. It is certainly worth exploring the effect of stopping smoking if you are contemplating hysterectomy for menstrual pain.

Drug Treatment

One effective treatment for menstrual pain is the group of drugs called anti-prostaglandins, which are successful in about 75 per cent of women. The drugs should be taken up to twelve hours before the occurrence of severe pain, so the tablets are best started the day before menstruation begins, or at the first sign of menstruation.

These drugs are more effective than other simple analgesics.

What is Pain?

The word 'pain' is derived from a Greek word meaning penalty. Although pain is a universal phenomenon it is nevertheless difficult to describe. Pain is not synonymous with injury. Broadly speaking there are three components to pain: the first indicates that the source of the pain is harmful and could cause physical damage; the second is the behaviour or pattern of responses associated with the pain and which enable an outsider to recognize that you are in pain; the third component is the personal or private feelings of 'hurt'.

Psychological Factors in Pain

Psychological factors may cause pain and frequently add to its severity. They may also diminish or abolish pain even in the presence of extensive damage.

In order for pain to be experienced not only must the nerve pathway and the central nervous system be intact but the stimulus must be processed psychologically. A woman in a coma is not aware of pain from a fractured pelvis. Painful conditions are often treated with narcotic drugs which, although not affecting nerve fibre pathways, alter the state of consciousness and influence mood and the perception of pain. Soldiers seriously injured in battle, or sportsmen receiving major injury often report they felt no pain until hours later. Religious mystics can undergo experiences usually considered painful, such as lying on beds of nails or walking on burning coals, without consciously experiencing pain.

Threshold of pain varies greatly from one person to another. At one end of the spectrum are people who are congenitally indifferent to pain. There is an absence of specific pain receptors in the skin of these people. At the opposite extreme are people who have little tolerance for pain. In this group, psychological elements predominate.

It is also important to make the distinction between the two components of pain experienced: the sensory component and the suffering component. This distinction has come into prominence in recent years following studies of patients undergoing brain surgery for relief of intractable pain. These patients commonly reported that the pain was there as before but that it no longer concerned them. The pain that remained was the sensory pain, the suffering had been relieved. The separate consideration of the sensory pain from suffering pain is important practically as well as theoretically. For example, it appears that morphine reduced 'suffering' more than 'sensory' pain.

There are broadly three principal ways for psychological factors to be important in pain. First, there is pain caused by muscle tension, where the tension itself results from psychological causes. Second, there is a mechanism by which some unconscious anxiety is reduced by being 'converted' into pain. A most striking example of the illustration of pain as a symptom solving unconscious conflict is that of fathers who may act as if suffering from pains or lie in bed after their wives' childbirth, while their wives continue in their usual occupations. The third mechanism is rarer and is the occurrence of pain as a hallucination in a serious psychiatric illness, for example, schizophrenia.

Pain because of any of these psychological factors has certain common characteristics. Most often it affects the head as headache, and is usually felt on both sides. More than one site is frequently involved. It is usually continuous, although it fluctuates somewhat throughout most of the day but does not keep the patient awake at night.

Psychological factors frequently make the pain of a physical condition worse, by affecting the threshold and perception of pain.

Pain is a frequent symptom in psychiatric illness, such

as anxiety or depression. This sort of pain responds well to the treatment of the psychiatric illness.

If you do not wish to take drugs for menstrual pain or find them no help, psychological techniques can be used to alleviate pain. It may require five to twelve visits to a doctor, psychologist or physiotherapist to learn the technique. A popular method is behavioural therapy. This combines relaxation techniques and mental imagery to reduce sensitivity to pain. The degree of relief varies, but the average reduction of pain is about one-third. The techniques may be used in conjunction with drugs, either to improve pain relief or to reduce the dose of drugs used.

Physical Disease

It is important to exclude physical disease which may cause menstrual pain. A doctor determines this by physical examination and in some cases, by carrying out a small procedure called a laparoscopy, an operation enabling the doctor to view the pelvis through a small incision in the abdomen.

Surgical Treatment

Hysterectomy is rarely necessary for menstrual pain unless it is related to physical disease. Before such a radical step is taken, make sure that you have considered or tried various treatments, for example, the pill, anti-prostaglandins, and psychological therapy. Other surgical treatments such as dilatation of the cervix or cutting the nerves to the uterus may lead only to temporary improvement, and for this reason are not popular.

Other Therapy

Many other treatments have been used for menstrual pain: hypnosis, acupuncture, hot and cold baths, and anti-spasmodics. Although less commonly used, such treatments may be worth trying when pain is severe and should be discussed with your doctor.

EXCESSIVE MENSTRUAL LOSS

What is Excessive Bleeding?

Most women judge the severity of bleeding from previous experience. A change in menstrual pad use is the most common way for a woman to judge the amount of menstrual loss. An increase in pad usage from four to eight a day may not mean that the blood loss is severe enough to cause anaemia, a criterion often used by doctors to judge whether menstruation is excessive. This degree of loss may be important and indicate the development of hormone imbalance of physical disease in the uterus. As indicated in Chapter 1, however, many women have difficulty in accurately perceiving an increase or decrease in the amount of menstrual blood loss.

Apart from the amount of blood loss in a day, the duration of menstruation is also important. If the length of menstruation is doubled from three to six days it may be caused by a disease. In judging the length of menstruation, the usual length of menses for that person must be considered. For example, if a woman is bleeding for six or seven days a month, which represents one quarter of her life, a further prolongation of one to two days may be intolerable and socially unacceptable. Any bleeding of more than seven days is very uncommon, affecting about 1 to 2 per cent of reproductive women, and should indicate that something may be wrong.

Frequency

Heavy or prolonged bleeding occurs in about one in ten women. Although less common than menstrual pain, heavy or prolonged bleeding may lead to disruption of life for several days, or to anaemia, or it may indicate the onset of physical disease.

It is important to see a doctor when menstruation is

prolonged or heavy to exclude the presence of disease. Intrauterine contraceptive devices, fibroids, endometriosis, pelvic infection, and cancer are common causes of heavy or prolonged bleeding.

Curettage

When no physical disease has been found, various treatments can be considered. In excluding physical disease, the doctor most often will curette the uterus to make sure there is no disease inside the uterus. Although curettage is done mainly to establish a diagnosis, occasionally it has a curative effect. It is not certain whether this reflects the removal of the lining of the endometrium, or whether it is the result of the rest in hospital or psychological relief from the exclusion of a serious cause.

Drug Treatments

Hormone treatments may be tried. There are two basic types: combined hormone treatments, using both oestrogen and progestogen, and single hormone treatments using progestogen alone. Combined hormone treatment is very popular if contraception is required, and in the first instance the simple contraceptive pills are tried. If these fail, then larger dose contraceptive pills may be used. It is important to consider the dangers and side effects of the combined pill in pursuing this treatment, particularly if treatment is required for more than a few months. Those who are overweight, smokers, or aged over forty should weigh the risks of pill treatment against other therapies. The progestogen alone pill has the advantage of not using oestrogen, which is the hormone responsible for thrombosis, a possible serious complication of combined hormone therapy, but it has the disadvantage of having side effects such as weight gain and depression. If the progestogens are successful and no side effects occur, they can be used for a long time. This may help in avoiding hysterectomy.

Other drugs which are very helpful for excessive bleeding are the anti-prostaglandins, mefenamic and flufenamic acid. On average, anti-prostaglandins reduce menstrual loss by about one-half and may be the best initial treatment if the combined hormone pill is unsafe for you or you experience unpleasant side effects when using hormones. Anti-prostaglandins have very few side effects and can be used for long periods of time.

In a small number of women who have heavy bleeding and are not ovulating, ovulation may be stimulated by the drug Clomiphene and the bleeding relieved.

A new treatment for excessive bleeding is Danazol, a drug which may reduce or stop menstruation. It is still very expensive and has a small risk of causing increased hair growth.

Surgical Treatment

Bleeding is a very common symptom leading to hysterectomy, even in the absence of physical disease of the uterus. It is important to diagnose physical disease and bleeding disorders, and to try simple drug regimes before having a hysterectomy. Some women are averse to drug therapies or impatient with such management and providing they understand the risks of hysterectomy, they may prefer it. In the absence of physical disease of the uterus, it is difficult for the doctor to decide when hysterectomy is in your best interest. You should try to help make the decision by considering the risks of the operation and comparing this to the way in which your life is impaired by heavy menses.

PHYSICAL DISEASES

The most common physical diseases leading to hysterectomy are fibromyomata, endometriosis, pelvic infection, and cancer. More rarely the uterus may be damaged at the time of childbirth or curettage.

Fibromyomata (fibroids)

Fibroids are lumps of muscle or fibrous tissue which grow within the normal muscle of the uterus. They vary in size from small seeds to lumps as large as a football. Fibroids are very common and are thought to occur in about a third of women over the age of forty. Fibroids do not spread outside the uterus, and are not a form of cancer. For these reasons, fibroids do not always need to be removed. Fig. 6 shows the various ways fibroids may grow.

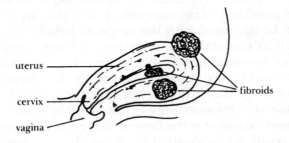

Figure 6 Diseases of the pelvic organs: fibroids

If fibroids cause heavy bleeding, menstrual pain, or are so large that they press on the neighbouring organs, the bladder, bowel or rectum, then it is best to have them removed. Occasionally, fibroids grow so large in the pelvis that sexual intercourse becomes difficult or painful.

The surgeon may advise the removal of large fibroids even though they are causing little or no effects, in the expectation that if they grow any larger, serious complications may occur and then removal is more dangerous.

Another factor which affects the decision about hysterectomy is the growth rate of fibroids. Normally, fibroids stop growing at the time of the menopause and thereafter either stay the same size or shrink. If the fibroids are small and first appear when you are between forty and fifty, and are causing no symptoms, it is likely that surgery will not be required.

Uncommonly, fibroids grow outwards from the womb, twist upon themselves and produce severe pain requiring urgent surgery.

Very rarely, fibroids may turn into a cancerous like growth called a 'sarcoma'. This is so uncommon as not to be a reason for always removing fibroids. If fibroids grow rapidly, however, the possibility of sarcoma has to be considered and would indicate surgery.

Sometimes fibroids can be removed (myomectomy) and the uterus repaired. If childbearing is still desirable, the possibility of myomectomy rather than hysterectomy can be discussed with the surgeon. Relief of symptoms such as menorrhagia or dysmenorrhoea is less reliable after myomectomy than hysterectomy. Sometimes myomectomy may be more dangerous than hysterectomy because of the difficulties in controlling blood loss. Occasionally, myomectomy is not possible as bleeding becomes excessive at the time of surgery and hysterectomy is required to control it. Fibroids may recur after myomectomy.

Unfortunately, no drugs will cure fibroids and as yet the cause of fibroids is unknown.

Endometriosis

This term is related to the word 'endometrium' which is the tissue lining the inside of the uterus. Endometriosis refers to endometrium existing outside its normal situation. It may occur in the wall of the uterus or outside the uterus, but is usually confined to the pelvis (see Fig. 7). It is thought to result from the endometrium spreading from the inner part of the uterus through the tubes, blood vessels or lymphatics or alternatively by normal cells elsewhere in the pelvis turning into endometrium. The disease is easy to understand if one realizes that the endometrium behaves very like the normal endometrium lining the inside of the uterus, growing during the menstrual cycle under the stimulation of the hormones from the ovary and then dying at the time of menstruation. The consequences of the cyclical activity (growth and dying) are necessarily different. Whereas the endometrium lining the uterus is shed as menses, the endometrium growing elsewhere in the pelvis cannot be shed, bleeds at the time of monthly dying, and may cause irritation, pain, or swelling in the tissue in which it exists. Blood cysts (fluid cavities) may then form on the ovaries or in any of the pelvic tissue overlying the bladder, bowel, or uterus. Each month the cysts become larger as more and more endometrial tissue develops and dies. The symptoms most commonly experienced are pain or disturbances of bladder or bowel function at the time of the periods.

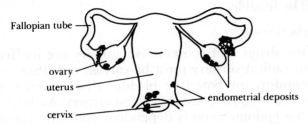

Fallopian tube

ovary

uterus

endometrial deposits

cervix

Figure 7 Diseases of the pelvic organs: endometriosis

Endometriosis has a variable course. It may cause no symptoms at all. On the other hand, it can be severely crippling, causing severe and recurrent pain.

The physical extent of the disease varies: it may affect only a small part of the pelvis, for example, one ovary; or it may extend over all the pelvic organs.

The duration of the disease also varies and it may occur only for one or two cycles or it may extend over the whole of the reproductive life.

Because of the variation in the severity of the disease and its natural course, no one treatment can be advised. The disease may burn itself out and disappear altogether so that no treatment is required.

There are three major methods of treatment: drugs, conservative surgery, and radical surgery.

Drugs

Hormones can be used to stop the growth of the endometrium which halts the spread of the disease and allows the diseased parts to heal. Drugs used are the combined oestrogen/progestogen contraceptive pills or progestogens alone. A new drug, Danazol, is the most effective.

Conservative surgery

If the drugs are ineffective, intolerable or infertility exists, conservative surgery may be better. The surgeon removes the diseased parts but leaves part or all of the pelvic organs so that menstruation and conception may still be feasible.

Radical surgery

If the drugs and conservative surgery are ineffective, then radical surgery must be carried out. Pain, sexual discomfort, or bowel or bladder dysfunction may be severe enough to consider radical surgery. As the growth of the endometrium is dependent upon the hormones made in the ovary, both ovaries are removed as well as the uterus and tubes.

Pelvic Infection

Infection in the pelvis is common. Fortunately, most infections are not serious. Those occuring at the entrance of or in the vagina are very common, a great nuisance, but not serious. Although proper treatment of these vaginal and vulval infections is important, they need not concern us as most of these infections do not spread to the uterus, tubes, or ovaries and therefore do not require surgical treatment. Less common but more serious are those infections occurring in the uterus, tubes, or ovaries. Such infections may lead to serious illness, infertility if the tubes are damaged, or to chronic pain and other menstrual upsets which may necessitate surgical removal of the organs involved.

Infections most commonly follow pregnancy, after either an abortion or childbirth. Infection may result from: venereal disease, usually gonorrhoea; the spread of infection from other organs, such as appendix or urinary tract, or via the bloodstream; toxic shock; intra-uterine devices; or more rarely tuberculosis or water skiing. The tubes are particularly susceptible to infection. Infections are best prevented, not treated. Good medical care during pregnancy and abortion, seeking medical advice whenever symptoms of pelvic infection are present, and avoiding venereal disease are all important.

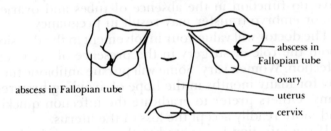

Figure 8 Diseases of the pelvic organs: infection of the Fallopian tubes

The most common symptoms of pelvic infection are abdominal pain, fever, and an offensive discharge. Sometimes menstrual disorders such as heavy or painful bleeding may be associated with the infection.

The best treatment of pelvic infections are antibiotics. These are given in high doses and repeated until all symptoms and signs of the infection have disappeared. This may involve a number of visits to the doctor as pelvic infection has a tendency to recur. After severe or recurrent attacks of infection, antibiotics may prove ineffective. It is hard to lay down exact rules, but it is worth treating pelvic infection with antibiotics for many months or even one or two years to try and stop the recurrent bouts of infection and also to clear up symptoms associated with the infection.

With severe or recurrent infections, the question of surgery may need to be considered. For example, severe bouts of infection may be life threatening. Alternatively, the recurrent bouts of infection may cause such pain and menstrual disorder that removal of the pelvic organs comes as a great relief. Once the tubes and ovaries are severely damaged and the disease persists, surgery is preferable.

Although the uterus is least affected by severe or recurrent infection it may have to be removed, as removing the tubes and ovaries alone sometimes leads to persistence of symptoms. While the uterus would appear to have no function in the absence of tubes and ovaries, donor embryo transfer may result in pregnancy.

The doctor will value your involvement in the decision about the role of surgery in the presence of recurrent infection. Women vary. Some will pursue antibiotic therapy for many months in the hope of avoiding hysterectomy. Others prefer to eradicate the infection quickly, and more readily accept the loss of the uterus.

If the infection has spread to the ovaries, it is almost certain that the surgeon will have to remove both ovaries with the tubes and uterus to be certain of curing the infection.

Cancer

Cancer of the uterus, tubes, and ovaries occurs in about three in every 100 women. Although cancer is not the most common reason for hysterectomy, it is a very important reason for hysterectomy because in many cases it is the only method of curing the cancer. The majority of women with uterine cancer are cured by treatment.

Uterine cancer occurs in two forms: an early or benign phase where the cancer cells have formed within the lining of the uterus but not spread anywhere, and a spreading phase where the cancer cells have spread into or outside the uterus.

In the early phase, when the cancer cells are still lining the uterus (non-invasive/pre-invasive cancer), an almost 100 per cent cure is possible. Treatments vary from removing the lining alone to removing the whole uterus. The lining can be removed with heat, by freezing or local surgery. Some doctors and patients prefer the uterus to be removed, particularly if the early phase cancer is extensive or has come back after previous removal or the patient has other reasons for uterine removal, such as severe menstrual symptoms or a dissatisfaction with repeated visits to gynaecologists to have cancer smears done.

When the cancer has invaded the uterus, hysterectomy is usually required. Tissue surrounding the uterus may also be removed, but the extent of the surgery will vary with the type and extent of the cancer. This is best discussed with the surgeon. Sometimes the upper part of the vagina may be removed but even after such an extensive operation, sexual function is possible. Treatments other than surgery may be given. Radiation, which kills cancer cells may be used. Drugs given as tablets or injections may also be used and after passing through the circulation may stop the growth of the cancer cells. Occasionally hormones also are helpful. Even in advanced cases of cancer, when cure is not possible, relief of symptoms and prolongation of life may be attained.

Cancer in the ovaries may spread to the uterus and if it does hysterectomy is required. In this instance, both ovaries are also removed.

Accidental Damage by Perforation at Curettage

Sometimes the uterus is perforated at curettage by one of the instruments used to carry out this procedure.

The perforation may be caused by a technical difficulty in carrying out the procedure or by the unusual shape or consistency of the uterus, making it more susceptible to perforation. Nearly always the hole in the uterus is small and heals without harm. After healing the hole does not affect subsequent menstruation. Rarely, bleeding may continue at the site of perforation and this may require surgery either to sew up the hole or, if the tear is large and bleeding is profuse, to remove the uterus.

Prolapse

Sometimes hysterectomy is carried out to assist in the treatment of prolapse. This may help in one of two ways. The uterus itself may be prolapsed or removal of the uterus may improve the repair of the muscle and ligaments supporting the vagina.

THE DECISION TO HAVE SURGERY

Both you and the doctor may find it difficult to make a decision about hysterectomy. Some women prefer the doctor to make the decision, some prefer to make the decision themselves, but most prefer an exchange of information and ideas whereby they and their doctor come to a mutual agreement about the best course of action. Except in life threatening situations the woman's view may influence the decision considerably. The woman's view depends upon three major factors.

The emotional value of the uterus is important and this will vary, depending upon the value placed on the production of menses, the need to conceive, and the possible role of the uterus in sexual function. The attitude of the woman to the physical risk and inconvenience of the disease and the operation will also be important, as will socio-cultural influences: the cost of surgery, the availability of skilled surgeons, the provision of adequate hospital facilities, and the peer and racial group attitudes to hysterectomy.

Some doctors find the involvement of the women confusing, particularly if the woman refuses hysterectomy when he or she thinks it is indicated. For example, a doctor was perplexed by a woman who had extensive cancer of the lining of the uterus (non-invasive) and who had completed her family size but wished to retain her uterus for sexual and menstrual reasons and elected to have local removal of the lining rather than hysterectomy. As long as the woman understands the risk of the disease, her decision concerning the treatment is an acceptable one. The doctor is responsible for giving advice and information which the patient may or may not accept.

Traditionally, the doctor has approached gynaecological surgery mainly from the viewpoint of physical risk. The woman may prefer a small physical risk in retaining the uterus in order to retain the emotional benefit of menstrual function. A decision about hysterectomy cannot be based solely on concepts of physical risk. The decision needs to take into account the emotional value placed on the uterus, the attitude to the physical risk of the disease and the operation, and the socio-cultural factors involved. When the emotional value of the uterus is low, physical dangers will determine the need for surgery, whereas, if the emotional value of the uterus is high, physical risks may be judged less important.

Situations may arise where the doctor considers that you have erred seriously in deciding for or against hysterectomy. Knowing you as a person and knowing the social factors influencing the decision may enable the doctor to counsel you to change your view.

If you are uncertain whether to have a hysterectomy, the decision can be delayed. It is often helpful to discuss the decision with your partner, a close friend, your general practitioner or, if you are still in doubt, a second specialist. Either the general practitioner or first specialist may refer you to a second specialist.

To summarize, a decision about hysterectomy will involve:

- an assessment of the physical risk of the gynaecological disease or symptoms
- a comparison of physical risks of various forms of

treatment

- an assessment by you of the emotional value of the uterus
- an assessment of emotional reactions to the disease and the operation
- an assessment of the social and cultural factors which may influence a decision
- an exchange of information between you and the doctor.

5 The Types of Hysterectomy and the Dangers

TYPES OF HYSTERECTOMY

There are different types of hysterectomy. The most common type of hysterectomy is total hysterectomy, where the whole uterus is removed. A subtotal hysterectomy is the removal of the body of the uterus but not the cervix. This is rarely performed but may be necessary when the cervix is difficult to remove and attempts at its removal may be dangerous. The main advantage in removing the cervix is the prevention of the risk of subsequent cancer of the cervix. Salpingo-oophorectomy refers to the removal of the tubes and ovaries and the uterus. This operation may be necessary when disease has spread to these structures, for example, severe infection, severe endometriosis, or cancer; where control of the disease may require removal of the hormonally active ovaries, for example, severe endometriosis; or in older women when the ovaries no longer function and removal stops the risk of ovarian cancer (see Fig. 9).

If you have cancer, a more extensive hysterectomy (Wertheim's extended hystectomy and lymphadenectomy) is required, the uterus, part of the vagina, and most of the tissues in the pelvis being removed. Complications are more common, but with advances in surgical technique, even this type of surgery produces few serious

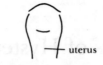

uterus

1 Sub-total hysterectomy

uterus

cervix

2 Total hysterectomy

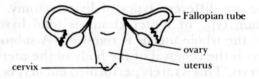

Fallopian tube

ovary

cervix

uterus

3 Total hysterectomy and bilateral salpingo-oophorectomy

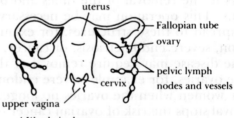

uterus

Fallopian tube

ovary

pelvic lymph
nodes and vessels

cervix

upper vagina

4 Wertheim hysterectomy

Figure 9 The various organs which are removed during the different types of hysterectomy

complications. The risk of damage to the ureter and bladder are slightly increased and the duration of convalescence prolonged.

If pre-invasive cancer exists in the top of the vagina and cervix the surgeon may remove the uterus and a small cuff (0.5 - 2.5 cm) from the top of the vagina. This involves more extensive surgery, but the risks are only slightly greater than those from total hysterectomy. The risk of damage to the ureter is slightly increased.

Method of Removal

There are two main avenues to the uterus: through the vagina or through the abdomen. Most surgeons operate through the abdomen. Greater skill is required to remove the uterus through the vagina unless the uterus has prolapsed down the vagina. The vaginal operation has the advantages of having one wound and avoiding an abdominal scar. If it is done by surgeons who are not skilled in the operation, however, it has a higher risk, in particular, there is a higher risk of bleeding. It is best to accept the type of hysterectomy recommended by the surgeon. If you are determined to have the vaginal operation, you need to ensure that the surgeon has the necessary skill and experience.

HYSTERECTOMY HAZARDS

Complications may occur during or after surgery.

Complications During the Operation

During the operation the surgeon may encounter difficulties which lead to damage to organs close to the uterus, the bladder and the tube going into the bladder (the ureter), the bowel and rectum.

Ureters

Recently, a woman successfully sued a doctor for negligence because both ureters were cut at the time of surgery. The ureters pass immediately next to the uterus on the side of the cervix. In order to avoid damage to these structures, the surgeon pushes the bladder away from the uterus and this carries the ureter away from the cervix so that clamps can be placed between the cervix and ureter to facilitate removal of the uterus and prevent bleeding. If the ureters are not displaced by the surgical technique, damage may occur. Even in the most skilled hands, the risk of damaging a ureter is about one in every 1000 hysterectomies. It is thought that the surgeon can avoid the ureter because the ureter can be seen or felt. This is not so. At the point where the ureter is most vulnerable, the ureter cannot be seen or easily felt. Even a full dissection of the ureter would not avoid the complication because the dissection itself may damage the ureter. The greatest assurance against damage to the ureter is to employ a skilled surgeon, but a one in 1000 risk of ureteric damage must be accepted. If the ureter is damaged, it is usually recognized and can be either joined together or replanted in the bladder. If it is unrecognized, further surgery will be necessary to identify the injury and repair the damage.

The bladder

The bladder is damaged more frequently than the ureter, but it is more easily recognized and dealt with. The risk of a surgeon making a hole in the bladder would be about one in 500. If it is recognized, the surgeon closes the hole in the bladder and healing follows. In this situation it may be necessary to rest the bladder by introducing a tube (catheter) into the bladder to drain the urine for a week after surgery. The bladder injury may not be recognized because sometimes the edge of the bladder is difficult to distinguish from the surrounding tissue and a stitch is placed in the bladder which subsequently dissolves, leaving a hole. In such a case, sometime after the operation, urine will flow from the bladder through the top of the vagina. This is called a fistula. Sometimes the hole closes when the bladder is drained by a catheter. Bladder injury may occur even with a highly skilled and experienced surgeon. If a fistula is established and does not heal spontaneously, it is important to obtain the service of a skilled surgeon to repair the hole. Only a small number of surgeons have experience in closing fistulae. It is worthwhile obtaining their services if this complication occurs.

The bowel
Damage to the bowel is less common. During dissection of adhesions between the uterus and bowel, a hole may be made in the bowel. Damage also may occur when disease spreads from the uterus to the surrounding bowel (intestine or rectum), for example, in severe infection, endometriosis, or cancer. In these circumstances, the surgeon will repair the hole in the bowel, although if the bowel damage is extensive a portion of the bowel may need to be removed by a general surgeon. Sometimes damage to the bowel is not apparent until after surgery. The blood supply to the bowel is reduced by the operation, and the hole develops some days after the operation as the bowel wall dies. In this situation, an emergency operation would be necessary to repair the bowel wall.

Early Post-operative Complications (while in hospital)

Complications occur in one in ten to one in four patients having a hysterectomy. Most of these complications are not serious and resolve within ten days of the operation. Sometimes complications delay the return home, most often for only a few days.

Wound
Wound complications are the most common and consist of bleeding or infection. Haemorrhage may result in a collection of blood which causes pain and bruising, and resolves by the blood either being drained, reabsorbed or discharged through the edges of the wound. Some

surgeons routinely drain the wound with a plastic tube to prevent blood collecting. Infection is usually obvious because fever occurs and the wound is tender, swollen, and red. Antibiotics may resolve the infection but if not, pus will form and be discharged from the wound. Occasionally, pus will not discharge from the wound so a hole is made in the wound by the surgeon.

Thromboembolus (clot)

One of the most dangerous complications from any type of surgery is thromboembolism. Thrombosis means the clotting of blood within a vessel. After hysterectomy, thrombosis sometimes occurs in a vein in the pelvis or leg. If the thrombosis leaves the vein, it is swept along in the blood stream and lodges in the lungs blocking the circulation, when it is called an embolus. Although thrombosis is not a danger to life, the embolus is, because if blood flow through the lungs is seriously impaired, blood cannot receive the oxygen needed to maintain life. Embolism in the lungs occurs in one in 500 patients following hysterectomy.

There are many factors that may cause thrombosis and these are worth understanding because some can be prevented. Patients who are overweight or heavy smokers have an increased chance of thrombosis. If the operation is not urgent, consideration should be given to reducing weight and stopping smoking before surgery.

Use of the contraceptive pill also increases the risk of thromboembolism. It is best to stop the pill one month before surgery. By doing this you may expose yourself to the risk of pregnancy, and alternative contraception should be used. An early pregnancy would be removed at the time of hysterectomy, but there may be moral objection to this.

The surgeon can also help prevent thromboembolism. Slow blood flow through the limbs and elsewhere may cause thrombosis. The blood flow can be sustained during the anaesthetic by artificially stimulating the calf muscles to contract. This method is commonly used and does not cause harm. Another method of preventing thrombosis is to have injections which make the blood more fluid. These injections may have one disadvantage, they increase the chance of bleeding in the wound or at the operative site, but such collections are not dangerous when compared to severe thromboembolism. If you are a high-risk patient, overweight, a smoker, or you have had a previous thrombosis, the surgeon will probably order injections (e.g. heparin) to make your blood more fluid.

It is important for the patient to recognize the early signs of both thrombosis in the legs or embolus in the lung. If the diagnosis is made early, treatment can be given which nearly always prevents any catastrophe.

The signs of thrombosis in the leg are tenderness in the middle of the calf, swelling of one or other ankle, or increasing soreness of the calf on movement.

Warning of an embolus in the lung may be the occurrence of pain on breathing, a cough without phlegm (dry cough), shortness of breath, and soreness or pain in the chest. If any of these symptoms occur, contact the nurse or doctor. Thrombosis or embolism would prolong hospital stay by one or more weeks, depending upon the severity of the condition.

Pneumonia or lung collapse may occur after the operation, but it is less common with modern anaesthesia. It is important to avoid surgery if you have an upper respiratory tract infection (bad cold) as this may predispose you to pneumonia after the operation. It is also important to stop smoking one week before surgery. If this is impossible and you accept the greater risk of a lung complication, try to reduce the number of cigarettes smoked each day. Breathing exercises before and after the operation and general body movements will help prevent complications, both those in the lung and from thrombosis. Adequate relief of pain, confidence that you will do no harm to yourself when you move, breathe, and cough, the help of a physiotherapist, and the avoidance of smoking all reduce the risk of lung complications.

Bladder

You have already learnt how close the bladder and bowel are to the uterus. During hysterectomy the bladder is dissected from the uterus and may suffer some bruising as a result. This may cause pain, particularly when the bladder is full or emptied. In addition some of the nerves and blood vessels running to the bladder are cut. Bruising or nerve damage may cause difficulty in emptying the bladder. This is usually overcome by the passage of a tube (catheter) into the bladder, usually only once. Rarely, the bladder may be rested for several days by the use of a catheter which drains the urine continuously into a closed bag beside the bed.

Because of the need to empty the bladder before the operation and perhaps as a result of dissection close to the bladder, bladder infections may occur. The symptoms are scalding when the urine is passed, and frequency (urine being passed more often than normal). Infections can be cleared by the use of antibiotics. The dissection or bruising of the bladder may also cause pain when passing urine, but there will be no scalding as the urine flows. If bladder function is abnormal immediately after surgery, the doctor will check for infection by sending the urine to the laboratory for examination.

The bowel

The most common but least serious complaint relates to bowel function. For about one day after hysterectomy, the bowel is less active than usual as a result of anaesthesia or manipulations during surgery or both. This is the reason why food is not given and fluids are restricted for a short time (four to twenty-four hours) after surgery. As soon as bowel activity starts, fluid intake can be increased and a light diet started. This is when patients suffer some distress from the bowel. The bowel increases its activity, but the mechanism associated with emptying of the bowel has not fully returned. Colicky pains occur, which are commonly referred to as wind pains. These increase in intensity until some wind (flatus) is passed after which the wind pains decrease. Wind pains may last for one to three days. Tactics to overcome wind pains vary. Pain relief may take the form of tablets such as Panadol or aspirin (analgesics) or in severe cases, injections such as pethidine, morphine, or Omnopon (narcotics). Codeine is probably best avoided as it may cause constipation. An old-fashioned remedy, charcoal tablets, absorb gas in the bowel, reducing distension and colic. Other treatments are laxatives, which stimulate the bowel or expand faeces, or the use of suppositories or enemas, which empty the bowel from below. Nurses, doctors, and patients have personal preferences in the use of laxatives, suppositories, and enemas. If you are particularly averse to any of the treatments, you should say so. Sooner or later the wind passes through the bowel and relief follows. Our own preference is for a mild laxative and if difficulty persists, a suppository. Strong laxatives and enemas are used when there is prolonged delay in emptying the bowel, particularly if this is associated with colic.

Very rarely, the bowel may be paralysed for a prolonged period of time following surgery. In this case you will be fed intravenously by fluid in a bottle which is run into a vein in the arm until the bowel recovers.

Very rarely, the bowel becomes blocked off a week or two after surgery because of an adhesion (chewing gum-like material) forming either between pieces of bowel or between the bowel and the site from where the uterus was removed. If the bowel is rested, the blockage may resolve but if not, further surgery is required. This is a rare and unpleasant complication requiring another operation, but the outcome is excellent.

Late Post-operative Complications
Late complications are things that go wrong after re-

turning home. Occasionally, a wound infection or blood collection does not become obvious until after leaving hospital. The doctor should be contacted to see if treatment is required. Often the infection will resolve with an antibiotic, and swelling from a blood collection will absorb itself.

Chest, bowel, or bladder problems usually occur before leaving hospital — but you may notice that both bladder and bowel function are different from before the operation. Soreness when starting micturition may result from a bruise on the bladder. Scalding when passing urine may mean an infection has occurred and the doctor should be contacted. Constipation may occur and changing the diet to eating more fruit and vegetables or a mild laxative may help. Occasionally, piles cause a problem. If pain or bleeding occurs with your motion, contact the doctor. Because of bruising, damage to nerves, or changes in anatomy following hysterectomy, bladder and bowel function may not be completely normal until one to two months after surgery.

It is important to realize that the rate of physical recovery from surgery varies greatly. Two examples illustrate this. One woman, the day after hysterectomy, helped make beds in the hospital ward. She left hospital five days after surgery, was doing all the housework a few days later, and was swimming and riding three weeks after surgery. Another woman was unable to leave bed until fourteen days after hysterectomy. She convalesced slowly at home and finally returned to work thirteen weeks after hysterectomy. Neither of the patients had post-operative complications. The variation in the physical recovery of the two patients demonstrates why it is difficult for a surgeon to give a fixed schedule for post-operative recovery. A fixed schedule has the disadvantage of making recovery too slow for some and too quick for others.

The main principle to remember is that when the wound is healed no physical harm can occur by increasing physical activity. You are the best judge of what to do. The mind and body will usually indicate what you are capable of doing. If you wish to walk, do so. If you can't cope, then rest more. When you can walk easily, try a new activity requiring a little more physical exertion.

There are two important matters to consider. Physical help in the home may help recovery. If this is not readily available, you may obtain help in the home from the local council or some other organization. Husbands, children, and relatives can be enlisted to help.

An important decision to make is when to drive. Emergency braking requires quick reflexes and strong physical action. When you can do the gardening or walk up stairs quickly, you are probably fit to drive.

Another late complication is vaginal discharge. The wound at the top of the vagina takes longer to heal than the abdominal scar. The reason is that the vagina is moist and bacteria grow more frequently and as a result healing is slower. Vaginal discharge varies in colour: red, brown, yellow, and white. Blood (red or brown) may be discharged from the vaginal wound. A yellowy smelly discharge indicates infections. The infection may heal naturally or with the help of antibiotics. The discharge usually disappears two weeks after surgery but sometimes lasts for six to eight weeks. If the discharge is prolonged beyond this time, the doctor should be notified. Sometimes a small amount of flesh forms on the edge of the wound. This is removed by burning with diathermy which is painless.

Once the vaginal wound is fully healed and emotional and physical recovery is advanced, sexual intercourse is resumed. Many women are nervous about intercourse because of fears of pain, pressure on the scar, or of causing internal damage. Once the wound is healed (no discharge) and the surgeon has examined the scar with a finger, coitus is possible. At the time of first intercourse it is worth telling your husband, if the doctor has not done this, that you are nervous and that it is important to be gentle. Deep penetration should be slow and gentle. If you wish to have intercourse but find deep thrusting uncomfortable, most men can climax without deep thrusting by moving the penis up and down in the lower part of the vagina. Vaginal scars are sometimes tender and it may be three months before the vaginal scar is flexible and not tender. Thus coital compromise may be necessary for two or three months.

If you and your husband both wish to have sexual satisfaction, but it is too early to have vaginal intercourse, or this is uncomfortable, then extra-vaginal sources of sexual satisfaction can be used, for example, masturbation or oral sex.

It is common for women to temporarily lose sexual feeling as a result of disease, surgery, and the post-operative experience. You should explain this to your husband and if necessary enlist your doctor's advice in helping to cope with the problem. Providing you enjoyed sex before the operation and you have recovered emotionally and physically, sexual desire will return. Your husband may help by not making sexual demands. Alternatively, you can tell him that you are happy for him to relieve his sexual drive by masturbation or you may help him to masturbate.

Prevention of Complications: your contribution

You can contribute to the reduction of physical dangers of hysterectomy. The check list includes selecting a skilled surgeon, reducing your weight if you are obese, reducing or stopping smoking, avoiding surgery if you have another illness and the operation is not urgent, stopping the oral contraceptive pill a month before surgery, and notifying the doctor of any medical diseases or drug allergies before undertaking the surgery.

Death

It is unlikely that a fit young or middle-aged woman would suffer death from hysterectomy, but even a very small risk must be considered in deciding on the need for surgery.

Death following hysterectomy is uncommon, occurring in one in 1000 to 3000 women. Most of the deaths occur in women who are elderly or obese or who have cancer or a medical disease such as high blood pressure. The deaths are caused by thromboembolism (blood clotting in the veins), haemorrhage, infection, anaesthesia, and coincident medical diseases. The risks of death from haemorrhage or anaesthesia may be reduced by having a skilled surgeon and anaesthetist in a properly equipped hospital, although even in the most skilled hands occasional complications occur.

Thromboembolism has been reduced in recent years because of preventive techniques. During the surgery, the calf muscles are stimulated to contract and this helps maintain blood flow through the limbs which prevents blood clot formation. In addition, injections can be given to make the blood more fluid to again prevent clotting. Patients who are at high risk of clotting, such as the obese, heavy smokers or women with previous thrombosis are given injections of anticoagulants to make the blood more fluid.

During surgery the patient's heart rate and blood pressure are checked so that any complications can be quickly detected and corrective action taken.

6 Emotions: Coping with your Feelings

EMOTIONS OR FEELINGS

Emotion refers to a person's subjective experiences, her perception of her inner emotional state and observable behavioural patterns that accompany these feelings. The fundamental or basic emotions include happiness, sadness, anger, and fear. Anxiety and depression are complexities of the basic emotions of fear and sadness. Clinically, anxious and depressive illnesses are greater in intensity and more prolonged in duration than the anxiety and depression we all experience from time to time.

It is important to realize that anxiety is a normal emotion and, within certain limits, is very helpful. It motivates you to do things: to be on time, to complete tasks. It is when anxiety is too high and too prolonged and interferes with your normal coping mechanisms and causes distress that it may be called pathological or clinical anxiety.

Feelings about the Operation

Hysterectomy may be necessitated by physical illness but sometimes an emotional disorder leads a woman to seek a hysterectomy. An example is the woman with a cancer phobia, where no amount of examination or reassurance can overcome her high anxiety and belief that she has a malignant disease. An operation rarely removes her phobia, which may occur as part of a severe depressive illness or may be part of a more general disease or body phobia. Excessive concern about the function of internal organs and multiple complaints may arise in a person with hypochondriasis. Pain may be of psychological origin, indicating inner distress. Very occasionally, people suffering from major psychiatric illnesses, such as schizophrenia, may go to their doctor with a bizarre preoccupation and over-concern which may lead them to a gynaecologist requesting hysterectomy. For most of those women surgery has little to offer. Indeed, it may reinforce their maladjusted ways of avoiding conflicts and handling anxiety.

Most women have some anxiety about having a surgical operation. With all surgery there are fears of damage, loss, destruction, dependency, and death. Fears of damage, loss, and destruction are quite common even for women who consider hysterectomy necessary and seek surgery to alleviate their symptoms. This damage may be seen in such terms as 'I will never be the same again'; I will grow fat and old and unattractive'; 'My sex organs will be different or impaired or raw inside for a long time'; 'I will grow old sooner'. Fears may exist that the bladder and bowel may be damaged by the operation causing loss of control. Some women fear that the operation will have a bad effect on their sexual relationships, making them no longer attractive to their partners or husbands; others are anxious about possible hormonal changes and the effects these will have on their appearance, skin, hair growth, sensitivity, and confidence.

Potential feared losses vary among women but include loss of 'the monthly badge of femininity' (i.e. menstruation); loss of childbearing ability; and loss of sexual and other capabilities. By far the most important loss for some women following the operation of hysterectomy is the permanent loss of childbearing capacity. Some women feel they are not proper women when they are unable to have any more children. Even women who have more children than their ideal or wished for family may feel a real sadness or sense of loss. Women who have no children at all, who consider they have failed in their child-bearing needs, for example, through miscarriages or still births, may be especially threatened by hysterectomy. This loss is the ultimate because they will never ever again conceive or give birth to a child.

On the other hand, the release from the fear of pregnancy, of further children, may be significant in a very favourable adjustment to the operation for some women.

Other anxieties at the time of the operation include fears of death, anaesthetics, helplessness, dependency, and destruction. Many women have difficulty in changing from being the person in the family on whom all were dependent to becoming a patient and being dependent on doctors and nurses.

Guilt and shame may be difficult fears for a woman to admit and discuss openly. Some may see the operation as a punishment. Guilt may be related to masturbation, previous abortion, giving birth to a defective child, extra-marital activities or because a woman had had 'too active a sex life' or 'had had sex too young'. Shame may not be admitted, but women may say they are not well rather than tell others the nature of the operation for fear that they will be labelled 'one of those'.

COPING WITH FEARS

You need to analyse your thoughts, beliefs, fears, and expectations of the operation. What does hysterectomy mean to *you*? You may be helped in clarifying your ideas by discussing your feelings with another person, such as your doctor. If you have difficulty in talking about feelings you may find it easier to write an essay to yourself on your feelings about the operation.

Compare your fears with the actual effects of the operation. Use this book to provide the basis for your knowledge of actual effects. If you have a specific fear that is not dealt with in this book, discuss it with your doctor. Comparison of fears with reality will lead you to discard fears that have no basis. Some anxieties are not easily discarded even when they are known to be irrational. These anxieties are often triggered by previous traumatic experiences or personality vulnerabilities. Talking with a professional skilled in psychological counselling may help you resolve these concerns before the operation.

Many women at this time are given unhelpful comments from 'friends' or relatives which tend to exacerbate anxieties. How do you deal with such remarks? Reply to the person that their comments amount to 'old wives tales' and have no substance. Your knowledge of the effects of the operation will place you on a firm footing here. You should inform your 'friend' that his or her remarks are unhelpful and likely to give women without your knowledge groundless anxiety. They should desist from making such harmful statements.

EMOTIONS FOLLOWING HYSTERECTOMY

For many women the operation of hysterectomy is a significant psychological and physical stress. Studies of people experiencing similar stress have demonstrated a pattern of response. Initially much of the associated painful feelings are blocked out and only gradually does the person allow aspects to surface and reach consciousness. The early response of many hysterectomy patients exemplifies this response to stress. Immediately after the operation there is often determined cheerfulness. From six weeks to six months after the operation many women experience frequent bouts of anxiety and sadness with wide mood swings. Most women are able to deal effectively with this stress. As painful thoughts gradually intrude to consciousness they are dealt with rationally with the support and encouragement of close relatives and the   doctor. The pattern of response to the stress of hysterectomy then is as follows:

Protest
'Oh no, it can't be true'
Denial
'Nothing has changed'
Painful thoughts
'I am defective, unloveable.'
Dealing with painful thoughts
'I am changed but not my basic identity.'
Outcome
'I will get on with life.'

This is the pattern followed by many women, and it leads to a positive adjustment to the operation.

Follow-up studies, twelve to eighteen months after hysterectomy show that many women have persisting psychiatric problems. It is important to note that over 75 per cent of the psychiatric problems occurred in those women who had psychiatric illness before the operation. As discussed in Chapter 1, of women about to undergo hysterectomy about 55 per cent have significant psychological problems.

Nevertheless, the operation of hysterectomy itself does precipitate depression in some women. Hysterectomy is a major procedure, presenting a considerable stress to the body, and requiring both physical and psychological re-adjustments.

WOMEN AT RISK OF PSYCHOLOGICAL POST-OPERATIVE PROBLEMS

Some women do not deal as well with the stress of hysterectomy. These women are likely to be those who have had previous poor response to stress. Women with pre-existing psychological problems are most at risk. A past history of any psychiatric treatment is also a risk factor, possibly indicating poor adjustment to stress in the past. The most frequent post-operative psychological problem was that of depression. Depression is known to occur as a reaction to a perceived loss. For example, most people feel depressed after a bereavement. It follows then that women who perceive hysterectomy as a loss will be more likely to become depressed. The 'losses' may be those of reproductive ability or because the woman feels she has somehow lost part of her femininity through the operation.

Another important risk factor is that of the 'unhelpfulness' or lack of support experienced by the woman at the time of operation from members of her family or friends. She may have felt let down by someone she expected to visit, been offered unhelpful, unwanted, and usually incorrect advice or met with little understanding or help from her husband. Some women find being in hospital difficult because it makes them dependent on others. This is likely to be more difficult for those who were not allowed to be dependent when young, for example, because of cool relationships with parents.

Unresolved anxieties about the effects of hysterectomy may lead to emotional problems after the operation. These are principally the conditions of anxiety and depression.

ANXIETY

Anxiety is an emotional experience which we have all encountered. Anxiety of a certain degree is a normal phenomenon, and serves a useful function by enhancing effort and alertness, and by helping to maintain high standards of work and behaviour. Anxiety involves two distinct components: a subjective experience, and a pattern of behaviour observed in others as well as in yourself. Pathological or clinical anxiety refers to the occurrence of anxiety of such severity, frequency, or duration that it interferes with well-being or efficiency.

A woman suffering from anxiety may have a tense apprehensive attitude, with increased muscle tension being shown in the facial expression and posture. She has difficulty in relaxing and sits on the edge of the chair during the interview, jumping at sudden noise. Tremors may be visible if muscle tension is marked. The eyes tend to be wide open and the pupils dilated. The patient may lick her lips because her mouth tends to be dry. Other bodily symptoms include aches and pains, and sweating, particularly the palms, armpits, and forehead. Tachycardia or fast pulse, palpitations, increased blood pressure, and peripheral vasoconstriction (pallor) of the hands and feet give rise to the typical pallor and cold extremities, whereas the arterioles of the blushing area of the neck and upper chest are usually dilated. Anxious women tend to have shallow breathing, sometimes with sighing respiration. Occasionally, appetite is impaired but more usually over-eating occurs. A woman may complain of being anxious, feeling nervous and tense, and sometimes she will tell what she is afraid of, for example, her fear of being alone, fainting in a large crowd, or crossing an open space, her difficulty in speech, or feeling generally uncomfortable with strangers and authority figures, younger colleagues outsmarting her, and so on. Sometimes the woman is suffering from 'free floating' anxiety, a feeling of impending disaster, or fearful anticipation, or a worry that she is going 'mad'.

Other women do not go to their doctor with obvious expressions of anxiety, but complain of bodily symptoms such as tension headaches, pelvic pain, facial pain, constriction or pain in the chest, muscle pains and aches, muscle stiffness, palpitations, or gastrointestinal symptoms. A woman may actually be convinced that she is suffering from some dreaded disease. Anxiety may be increased because of painful conditions, or may be an exacerbating factor and increase pain.

Treatment of Anxiety

There are no easy rules to cover all the clinical problems of anxiety. It is well known that medication alone is not a complete answer. All women should receive time to discuss their anxieties and their feelings with an understanding, tolerant doctor who at least attempts to 'get inside the skin' of the patient and understand her. It would seem that too frequently the short-cut is to prescribe an anti-anxiety agent or drug rather than to help the person to understand and cope with her anxiety.

In longer standing anxiety, the treatment aims are twofold. The more severe manifestations of anxiety and associated depression—phobic symptoms or fears, unreal feelings, and panic attacks—need to be brought under control by measures aimed directly at the disabling symptoms. Some attempts should also be made to help the person acquire some understanding of the vulnerable facets in her personality that have contributed to her anxiety, and the manner in which they have arisen.

Although no specifically effective treatments exist, there are a number of measures that will bring relief of symptoms. These may be broadly grouped as psychological and physical therapies. The psychological measures include psychotherapy or counselling, relaxation techniques, and medical hypnosis principles. Few experts recommend any drug as sole therapy for the management of anxiety.

DEPRESSIVE ILLNESS

The important depressive symptoms are sleep disturbance, tiredness, loss of interest, and the depressed mood itself, with the accompanying depressive thoughts such as self-blame, difficulty in concentration, painful and suicidal thoughts, anxiety, irritability, paranoid ideas, retardation, and aches and pains.

The facial appearance of most depressed patients is characterized by furrowed brow, immobile face, downturned mouth, and an expression of troubled perplexity. Stooped posture and slow movements or restless agitation are important signs.

Depressive illness may be precipitated by a number of factors, including physical illness or operations. The actual cause is still unclear. Biochemical theories suggest some depletion of certain chemicals within the central nervous system. Family and twin studies have shown a genetic predisposition to depressive illness. Psychological theories emphasize loss: loss of physical health or capabilities, loss of status, loss either real, threatened or imagined in some people with certain personality structures.

Mild depression, the largest group, requires psychological treatment. Moderate depression is usually treated with antidepressant drugs and counselling. Severe depression usually responds to electroconvulsive therapy (shock treatment).

POST-OPERATIVE SEXUAL OUTCOME

Many women fear that hysterectomy will affect their sex lives. A German study found that two-thirds of the women interviewed expected a loss of feeling during intercourse and half expected their capacity for orgasm to be affected by hysterectomy. In our own study we found that 42 per cent of women interviewed after their operation had expected that the operation would impair their sex lives. These anxieties sometimes arose because of lack of knowledge of sexual anatomy or followed unhelpful comments from friends. In others such fears followed ideas that their feminine identity was altered by the operation.

How justified are these expectations? What percentage of women experience a deterioration in their sex lives? To answer these questions adequately it is necessary to draw once again on the results of studies in which women were assessed both before and after operation. These studies suggest that on the whole sexual relationships improve after hysterectomy. This is not surprising because before the operation sexual relationships would probably have been impaired by symptoms such as bleeding or pain. These symptoms are usually alleviated by the operation. A Sydney study found that after hysterectomy sexual relationships were reported as better by

55 per cent, unchanged by 28 per cent, and less satisfactory by 16 per cent. In the US study, 88 per cent reported an increase or no change in the frequency of sex and 12 per cent a decrease at the twelve-month post-operative visit. A New Zealand study reported similar findings with only 12 per cent experiencing a reduction in desire for sex and 6 per cent reporting less sexual activity.

The actual incidence of deterioration in sexual relationships following hysterectomy is a small one when women are assessed both before and after surgery. Interestingly, when women are interviewed only *after* the hysterectomy, a much larger percentage (37 per cent in our study) attribute their sexual problems to the operation.

WOMEN AT RISK OF A POOR SEXUAL OUTCOME

Women with negative expectations of how the operation will affect their sex lives are especially likely to develop sexual problems after the operation. In such cases their expectations are fulfilled.

Also at risk are women with other psychological problems, such as depression, which may impair the relationship with their partner.

Those women with a poor relationship with their sexual partner at the time of hysterectomy, when helpful supportive relationships are needed, are also liable to develop sexual problems. Although sexual problems which reflect gynaecological disease can be expected to improve after hysterectomy, women with a poor sexual adjustment before the operation are unlikely to be helped by the operation.

Fears of sexual and emotional consequences of hysterectomy abound, but the risk is small. Women most at risk of sexual or psychological problems after the operation are those who had such problems before the operation, who had expectations of being altered sexually or in their femininity by the operation, and who experienced a lack of support from their husband or partner or other friends or relatives.

7 Practicalities: Before, During and After Surgery

COMMON QUESTIONS

Women and men ask many questions about hysterectomy. Here are answers to the most common ones.

What fills up the hole when the uterus is removed?
Women often wonder whether an empty space remains in the abdomen. The answer is no. The bladder, bowel, and intestine take up the space. (See Fig. 10.)

Will hysterectomy ruin my sex life?
No. There will be temporary dislocation of sexual life as discussed in detail in Chapters 3 and 6. If sex is good before surgery, it should be good after surgery. If you had sexual difficulties before surgery, surgery may compound the problem further, and you may need special counselling.

Will hysterectomy upset my ovaries and lead to premature menopause?
No. Usually, the ovaries continue to function as the blood supply of the ovaries comes from a different source from the uterus. Rarely, the blood supply to the ovaries is impeded by thrombosis, and could lead to premature ovarian failure. This can be overcome by hormone therapy. (See Chapter 8.)

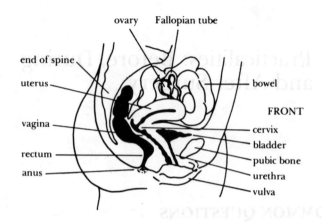

(a) Before hysterectomy

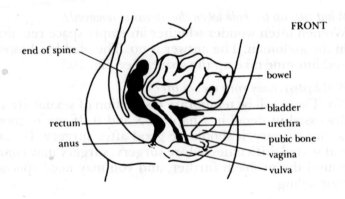

(b) After hysterectomy

Figure 10: Cross-section of the body showing position of the pelvic organs before and after hysterectomy

Will my hair fall out?
After any type of surgery temporary changes in the hair are common. Some women notice that their hair seems

dry and more falls out, but this is a temporary phenomenon.

Will my skin go wrinkly and dry?
No. If the uterus is removed, there is no permanent effect on the skin. After any operation a temporary change in the skin may occur. If the ovaries are removed then some women do notice skin changes, such as dryness but this can be overcome by hormone treatment. Hormone therapy is discussed in Chapter 9.

Will I age prematurely?
No. You may feel older while you are recovering from the operation because of the reaction to emotional and physical stress, but once you have fully recovered you will feel your usual self.

Will I be less attractive to my husband?
No. There will be a temporary period when you are recovering from surgery when you will not be so physically attractive, but once you have recovered your physical appearance will improve again.

Will hysterectomy affect my work?
Any change should be temporary. The effects of surgery, anaesthetics, and drugs may make it difficult to concentrate for some weeks. This should be taken into account when deciding to return to work. If your work is predominantly physical, your physical condition will determine when you can be effective again. Alternatively, if you are predominantly a mental worker, assessment of your intellectual and emotional condition is more important.

What danger is the operation to me?
This has been defined in Chapter 5. The risk is very small. Among survivors there is the bonus of avoiding the risk of death from cancer of the uterus. Only you can answer the question of whether the risk is worth the possible benefits from surgery.

How long do I need to be off work?
This varies. Employers like to work on a fixed time schedule. On average, women are off work for six weeks, but it is best for you to negotiate a variable time period with your employer because you may be fit for work as early as three weeks after surgery or you may not be fit for work until ten weeks after surgery.

How long will I need to be in hospital?
On average, seven days, but this varies from five to fourteen. If complications occur, it may be prolonged.

What can I do when I go home?
The principle is that you will not harm yourself providing you let your own emotional and physical condition determine what you do. Increase your activity gradually. Most women do little in the first week after returning home but resume light housework and start more strenuous activities after this. Physical exercise is good because once the wound is healed (seven to ten days) abdominal exercises improve both the strength of the abdomen, which has been weakened by the surgery, and the comfort of the scar.

How much pain will I have?
There are two common types of pain: the pain from the wound, which is most severe on the first day or two after surgery, and the pain from the bowel, which is most severe from the second to fourth day after surgery. The severity of pain varies with the individual. The pain will be reduced by injections or tablets.

Will I have an intravenous drip?
Some surgeons use an intravenous infusion of fluid in all patients, but this is usually discontinued the day after surgery as soon as you can keep fluids down. The extra fluid reduces thirst and may speed recovery. The intravenous infusion system is also convenient if blood has to be given.

Can I have a hysterectomy through the vagina?
Often this is feasible, particularly if the surgeon is skilled in the vaginal technique. Most hysterectomies, however, are still done through an incision in the abdomen. The types of hysterectomy are described in Chapter 5.

Do I really need the hysterectomy?
If you are uncertain, you should seek a second opinion by consulting your general practitioner or by seeing another specialist. The decision-making process is descussed in Chapter 4.

Are there alternatives to hysterectomy?
You may feel that the surgeon advising you has not discussed alternatives to surgery and if so, you should obtain a second opinion. Alternative methods of treating many diseases are discussed in Chapter 4.

When could I have the operation done?
Most surgeons arrange the operation one to eight weeks after the decision has been made. If the operation is not urgent, you can plan to have it done at your convenience, for example, during school holidays. If your general health needs time to improve, it is important not to be impatient about having surgery because pre-operative preparation may reduce physical risks.

How much will it cost?
The costs include the fees of the surgeon, the anaesthetist, the assistant surgeon, the hospital, and the pathologist.

Do I need help when I go home?
For the first week some help is usually necessary and this can be given by your husband, children, or relatives. If there is no one you know who can help you, local council help can often be arranged with the aid of a doctor's certificate.

When can I drive?
When you can do light gardening or walk up the stairs

quickly. This usually occurs about three to six weeks after surgery.

When can I have sex?
When the vaginal wound is healed and you feel you wish to have it. The healing of the vaginal scar is checked by the doctor after surgery. The appointment can be made to suit you, should early return to sex be desired. (See Chapter 3.)

Will I injure myself by lifting things after surgery?
No. Most healing occurs within the first two weeks. After you have returned home, test yourself out lifting; providing your body feels comfortable, you will do no harm. There is a common myth that activities such as lifting or stretching to put clothes on the clothes line, for example, may undo stitches or weaken wounds. This is not so. Figures 11 and 12 show the correct and incorrect positions for lifting.

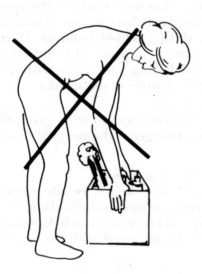

Figure 11 Incorrect position for lifting

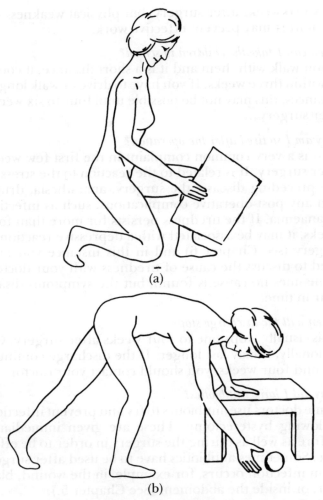

(a)

(b)

Figure 12 Correct positions for lifting

When can I do housework?
Usually light housework can be performed one to two
weeks after returning home. Sometimes it is not possible
to resume full housework duties until six weeks after
surgery. No harm will be done by attempting physical

work two weeks after surgery, but physical weakness or discomfort may prevent effective work.

When can I take the children to school?
If you walk with them and it is a short distance, it could be within three weeks. If you have to drive or walk longer distances, this may not be possible until four to six weeks after surgery.

Why am I so tired after the operation?
This is a very common complaint in the first few weeks after surgery. It is related to the reaction to the stress of the preceding disease, the surgery, anaesthesia, drugs, and any post-operative complications, such as infection or anaemia. If the tiredness persists for more than four weeks, it may be associated with a depressive reaction to surgery (see Chapter 6) and in this instance you may need to discuss the cause of tiredness with your doctor. Sometimes no cause is found, but the symptoms disappear in time.

When will the discharge stop?
This usually stops one to four weeks after surgery. Occasionally, it may last longer. If the discharge continues beyond four weeks, you should contact your doctor.

Why did I have antibiotics?
Some doctors use antibiotics to try and prevent infections following hysterectomy. These are given immediately before as well as during the surgery in order to be effective. Sometimes antibiotics have to be used after surgery if an infection occurs, for example, in the wound, bladder, or inside the abdomen. (See Chapter 5.)

CHOICE OF DOCTOR

Most often the general practitioner or family physician is consulted about a need for hysterectomy and he or she also can tell you when hysterectomy may be beneficial and also discuss who should do the surgery. The general practitioners have not been trained in general or gynaecological surgery and prefer to refer you to a specialist for the operation. If you are uncertain after visiting the gynaecologist whether you wish to have the operation, it may be helpful to have a further discussion with your general practitioner. If you are unhappy with the opinion of the gynaecologist, the general practitioner may refer you to a second gynaecologist for another opinion. The second opinion is often worthwhile because doctors sometimes disagree on the indications for hysterectomy. Doctors in New South Wales, Australia, for example, more often recommend the operation than in other Australian states. You may be placed in the position of having to decide between two expert opinions. You have the option of taking the opinion which suits your own inclination. Selecting a specialist is difficult because surgical skills for an operation such as hysterectomy are not easily measured.

There are four factors which are important in selecting a surgeon: whether or not you like the surgeon; the surgeon's ability to select patients correctly for hysterectomy; surgical skill; and clinical post-operative care and the cost. You have to rely on the general practitioner's opinion or perhaps the opinion of other patients who have been treated by the surgeon. Many patients are not offered the choice of a gynaecologist. In making a final decision you and your husband should discuss the matter. The opinion of friends may be helpful, but remember that if someone has an unpleasant experience following surgery it does not necessarily reflect on the clinical skills of the doctor. Although it is self-evident, remember that the fee charged, personality, and mode of dress do not reflect the skill of the surgeon.

TYPE OF HOSPITAL

After deciding to have the operation you make a decision whether to be a private or public patient.

One disadvantage of public hospital care is that you cannot choose the surgeon who performs the operation. It is unknown whether complication rates from trainee surgeons are higher than from experienced surgeons, although it is generally believed that this would be so. The trainee surgeons are supervised by more experienced surgeons. The other disadvantage of a public hospital is that you may be in a large ward with other patients. This suits some people but not others. One advantage of a public hospital is that if there is an emergency, modern equipment and medical specialists are quickly available.

The private medical system has the advantage of choice of an established surgeon and better conditions in hospital: privacy and comfort.

If you wish to have private surgery, you need to check to see if your health insurance payments cover the costs. If you are not insured and if the operation is not urgent, you can join a health insurance scheme, but you may need to pay the premiums for some months before you would qualify for repayment of costs.

When you go to hospital, it is important to know where to go and what to bring with you. Private hospitals may ask for evidence of health insurance or ask you to pay part or whole of the hospital fee, either on admission or before discharge. It is also helpful to provide the telephone number of your husband or next of kin which can be used by the surgeon or staff to convey information about your state of health after surgery or to help arrange your discharge from hospital.

DETAILS OF SURGERY

Many women have no idea what was found at operation. You should ask the surgeon if the uterus was normal. If it was not, ask what was wrong. A diagram of the abnormal uterus is helpful. It not only explains what has happened but also provides a record for any further medical consultations after surgery.

PRE-OPERATIVE PREPARATION

Blood may be collected from your ear or arm to establish your blood group because you may need extra blood during surgery. Most often blood transfusion is not necessary. Your haemoglobin level is measured which shows how much blood you have, and if the haemoglobin level is low, the surgeon may give you iron or blood before or after the operation.

The lower part of the abdomen is shaved as the incision needs to be free of hair so that it can be sewn satisfactorily.

Enemas or suppositories are not used routinely before hysterectomy, although they were popular some years ago. If you suffer from constipation or feel blown up, an enema before the operation may make your post-operative period more comfortable. It may be helpful to discuss your bowel function with the sister after admission to hospital.

Most patients are offered a sedative the night before surgery because the anxiety about the operation and the unfamiliar surroundings may make sleep difficult. You do not have to take the sedative if you feel you do not want to sleep or can sleep without the tablet. About half to one hour before surgery you are given an injection to facilitate anaesthesia and to avoid some of the complications that may occur during or after anaesthesia. Sometimes the surgeon will add other medications just before the operation such as antibiotics or injections to prevent thrombosis.

If you are prone to chest (pulmonary) complications, a physiotherapist may visit you before surgery and give you chest exercises to practise.

OPERATION

Patients are sent on a trolley from the ward to the operating theatre a short time before surgery. At this time you should be drowsy or at least feel at rest. Sometimes the drugs are less effective so that you may still be apprehensive. The anaesthetic is started outside or inside the operating theatre. You may feel anxious at this time but the staff try to help you relax and the anaesthetist starts the anaesthetic as soon as possible. Anaesthetics today start with an injection in a vein of the arm and going to sleep is a pleasant experience. Occasionally, the anaesthetist will have difficulty inserting the needle into the vein and several punctures of the skin may be necessary.

POST-OPERATIVE PERIOD

Experience of patients waking up after surgery varies. Some patients find breathing difficult. There is a nurse with you and if you have difficulty, an extra injection or an oxygen mask will be given until breathing is normal. The anaesthetist may see you again to make sure your breathing and general condition of health is satisfactory. Sometimes vomiting occurs immediately after anaesthesia. An injection will be given to stop or diminish the vomiting. Although most people feel relieved when first awake, some notice the pain from the wound and need an injection. A few women react by crying or being very talkative. There is no need for concern about how you will behave as staff are used to different reactions and anything you say is regarded as confidential!

Providing the observations of your breathing, pulse rate, and blood pressure are normal, you will return to the ward about one hour after surgery. If you have vomiting or pain, you will have been given drugs to help overcome this. You may notice a tube running to your arm; this is often a standard procedure, fluid running from a bottle into a vein of your arm.

The nurse or sister will see you at regular intervals during the first twenty-four hours after surgery, when you will be given injections for pain. It is sometimes difficult to find the correct dose or frequency of injection of a drug which gives effective pain relief. The longer you require injections for pain relief, the slower the post-operative recovery, because the drugs affect your ability to move or walk around. It is best to ask for injections when you feel you cannot cope with the pain but to change from injections to tablets (which are not as strong) as soon as possible. Pain often seems worse at night so that an injection in the evening is needed even when you can cope with the pain during the daytime. You may suffer mild withdrawal symptoms after stopping injections for pain. A mild depressive reaction may occur for a day or two. Most patients are feeling much better by the fourth or fifth day after surgery.

The rules concerning oral intake vary according to your condition immediately after the operation and your surgeon's beliefs. Some doctors encourage early drinking and feeding after surgery; others are more conservative. One matter is important: if you feel nauseated or have vomited, you should not be taking solid food. Tolerance of different fluids varies from patient to patient. For example, soon after surgery some patients can take water but not fruit juice and others prefer fruit juice or tea to water. If you are nauseated, favourite remedies such as lemonade or dry ginger ale may be best. When you first take food it will be a light diet consisting of semi-solids. Once you have coped with this, you will be able to have a solid diet, and providing you feel hungry you should try this. Some patients find their appetite has not fully recovered until after they have returned home. Antibiotics, narcotics, infection, pain, and depression all reduce appetite.

If you have an intravenous drip, you may suffer two problems: discomfort at the site of the needle or fear that air will run into the circulation when the drip runs out in the middle of the night. Discomfort at the needle site should be reported to the nurse because sometimes thrombosis or inflammation occurs and a new drip is needed. Providing there is no extra pressure in the intravenous system, such as when blood is being pumped under pressure (which is rare), there is no risk of air entering the circulation if the bottle runs out, but it is worth letting the staff know when the bottle of fluid is nearly empty so that the new bottle can be started.

It is best to be frank with the staff after surgery. If everything is going according to plan, at least as you see it, then obviously you need make no comment. But if you are worried or anxious, it is best to ask questions. Good medical care is helped by the co-operation and accurate observation of the patient.

ADVICE FOR THE FAMILY

Your partner and family are often confused about how to treat you after the operation. For example, if your husband is very 'understanding' and does not initiate sex in the months after the operation, you may fear that you are an invalid and no longer sexually attractive. If he treats you in exactly the same way as before the operation, making no concessions for the effects of major surgery, you may perceive him as callous and non-caring. How do women want to be treated at this time? Evidence of care, support, and helpfulness will help you to adjust to the operation and to increase the warmth and closeness in your own personal relationship. Questions about the speed at which you should return to physical activities should be discussed together, with your doctor, so that you have similar expectations. Your knowledge and understanding of the effects of the operation will help you to deal more effectively with the situation.

8 The Menopause

Men-o-pause literally means that menses stop. One meaning of menopause is the age at which the last period occurred. The other meaning of menopause is that of 'the change of life', the phase during which progressive failure of the ovaries occurs. The failure of the ovaries to produce hormones leads to the end of menstruation and other symptoms, such as hot flushes.

The usual time period during which menses stop for most women is between forty-five and fifty-five although 9 per cent of women are still menstruating at fifty-five. A few women experience menopause at a much earlier age (e.g. before they are forty) a condition known as premature menopause. These women are more likely to have had a late puberty, and there may be a family history of early menopause.

HYSTERECTOMY AND MENOPAUSE

Many women are confused about the relationship between hysterectomy and menopause. Frequent questions asked are: Will I experience one menopause or two? As I have already been through the menopause, will I now experience another? How will I recognize that menopause has occurred after hysterectomy? Will I need hormone replacement therapy after hysterectomy?

Much of the confusion is caused by the dual meaning

of menopause as both the time at which menses cease and the time during which there is ovarian failure. In the woman who is still menstruating, hysterectomy surgically halts menstrual flow by removing the source of the menses. But unless the ovaries are also removed the woman will not experience any symptoms from hormonal alterations until she reaches the stage of natural ovarian failure. She will thus experience two 'menopauses'. The first will be simply the ceasing of menses at the time of hysterectomy. The second will be the effects of ovarian failure when her ovaries reach the 'natural' menopause.

Sometimes the ovaries are removed at the same time as the uterus. This operation is known as hysterectomy and bilateral salpingo-oophorectomy. This may be necessary because of disease affecting the ovaries or for preventative measures (e.g. to halt the spread of cancer, see Chapter 5). The woman who has not yet reached a natural menopause will experience a sudden and severe menopause if both ovaries and uterus are removed. Menses will cease and symptoms of hormone deficiency will occur. Unless there are contraindications, most doctors prescribe hormones to replace those produced by the ovary. As the ovaries are now removed there will be no later menopause to undergo.

The postmenopausal woman who undergoes hysterectomy will not experience another menopause as her ovarian function and her menses have already stopped.

In order to understand and recognize menopausal changes and evaluate the role of hormone replacement therapy, it is necessary to consider the effects of the ovarian hormones and the hormonal changes which occur at menopause.

OVARIAN HORMONES

The ovaries lie one on either side of the uterus. They have two related functions: to manufacture hormones and to produce eggs.

At birth a female child has about 500 000 eggs. After puberty is reached, one or two of these egg cells or 'ova' are brought to maturity each month and released at the time of ovulation, which occurs about mid cycle. Throughout reproductive life (i.e. from puberty to menopause) these ova are depleted either by their release or by degenerative changes. Few egg cells are left at menopause.

The small cyst (or follicle) which brings the egg to maturity also produces chemical messengers or sex hormones. These hormones are called oestrogen and progesterone. As with other hormones, they travel in the bloodstream and have effects at sites in the body often a long way away from their points of origin. During a woman's reproductive life the amount of oestrogen and progesterone produced varies regularly in phase with the menstrual cycle.

Following each menstruation a new egg starts to mature within the follicle. This follicle also produces oestrogen in increasing amounts, reaching a peak at ovulation when the egg is released. The amount of oestrogen then falls temporarily. The follicle then starts to produce more oestrogen and progesterone, reaching a peak level of these hormones a few days before the next menstruation.

If the egg released at ovulation is fertilized and implants successfully in the uterine lining, a special messenger hormone will be sent by the egg. This hormone will notify the ovary of implantation, stimulate the hormone producing follicle to continue hormone production and thus maintain the uterine lining as a nutritious bed in which the fetus safely develops. This thick uterine lining or endometrium is produced by the stimulatory actions of both oestrogen and progesterone on the uterus. A new lining is produced each month in order to nourish a possible fertilized egg. Menstruation occurs because of the failure of the egg to enter this bed.

The development of the egg is influenced by the brain. The production of oestrogen and progesterone is controlled by the pituitary, a small organ lying at the base of the brain. The pituitary produces hormones which stimulate the follicles to develop. The pituitary is connected with many other areas of the brain and is directly influenced by brain function. Hormone production is shown in Fig. 1, Chapter 1.

As the follicles develop, ovarian hormones are produced which travel through the blood vessels to the brain and notify the progress that is occurring in the ovary. This important feedback from the ovary to the brain influences the amount of hormones produced by the pituitary.

Ovarian hormones have effects all over the body and particularly influence the growth and health of the genital organs. At puberty the sudden production of these hormones stimulates the growth of the breasts and the vulva (outer area surrounding the entrance to the vagina). Oestrogen has a stimulatory effect on the vaginal lining, causing an increase in thickness and pliability. Oestrogen increases the ability of the vagina to respond to sexual arousal with the secretion of a lubricating fluid. In addition, oestrogen also keeps healthy the lower part of the urinary tract and stimulates the growth of the uterus.

The pelvic muscles keep the uterus, urinary passage and bladder, and the lower part of the bowel in correct position. The tone and health of these muscles are maintained by oestrogen.

In addition to the monthly changes in the lining of the uterus, breast changes also occur each month. Many women are aware of an increase in size or fullness of the breasts premenstrually. These cyclical changes in the breasts are the result of the effects of oestrogen and progesterone on the glands of the breasts.

Oestrogen and progesterone also have more general effects. Oestrogen helps keep bones healthy and in particular helps maintain the thickness of bones. It is likely that the ovarian hormones have some protective effects on the blood vessels and heart.

In addition to the effects of ovarian hormones on the physical structures of the body there are influences on behaviour. During reproductive life most women are aware of mood fluctuations with the menstrual cycle. For most women favourable moods such as feelings of well-being and happiness occur most frequently in the early part of the menstrual cycle and at ovulation, a phase of increasing oestrogen.

There is an increase in irritability, tension, and depression in the latter part of the menstrual cycle, particularly in the last few days premenstrually. Although the causes of these changes are not clear, it is possible that they may reflect the changing oestrogen and progesterone balance. In some women these unpleasant moods are severe and called 'premenstrual tension'.

Oestrogen and progesterone also affect sexual behaviour. The influence of these hormones is more marked in animals where the role of social and psychological factors are less influential than in the human. Monkeys and apes have, like humans, a menstrual cycle. Experiments with these animals have shown clearly that oestrogen stimulates sexuality and progesterone is inhibitory, decreasing sexual responsiveness and attractiveness to the male. At first, studies of human sexuality found no consistent peak of sexual activity occurring in relation to the menstrual cycle. There was evidence of less intercourse during menstruation. A more recent study has examined female sexual desire and initiation of sex rather than the occurrence of intercourse which may not reflect the woman's own desire. This investigation suggests that there may be a cycle for sexual desire in human females with a peak occurring at mid cycle (high oestrogen) and a decline or trough corresponding to the production of progesterone.

HORMONAL CHANGES AT THE MENOPAUSE

The hormonal changes which occur at the menopause

are the result of the failure of ovarian function. Few egg cells remain, follicles do not develop, and the production of ovarian oestrogen and progesterone virtually ceases. This drop in the concentration of oestrogen and progesterone is noted by the brain which increases the amount of hormones secreted by the pituitary in an attempt to stimulate the ovaries and increase output of oestrogen and progesterone. This increase in pituitary hormones accurs with the approach of the menopause. Very high levels of these hormones are reached after the menopause. With increasing age the levels of these pituitary hormones diminish but usually remain higher than pre-menopausal levels. A simple blood test will enable your doctor to assess hormonal function. The amount of pituitary hormone (FSH) in the blood will indicate whether you are menopausal.

Other glands, such as the adrenal gland, may compensate partly for the failure of the ovary. Among the hormones that the adrenal produces are androgens. Androgens are sometimes called 'male' sex hormones even though they are produced in small amounts by all normal women. In men androgens are present in much larger amounts and produce the deep voice and hair growth pattern characteristic of males. Androgens can be converted to oestrogen by different parts of the body, including fat and brain cells. The amount of oestrogen produced in this way is variable, so that some women have more oestrogen than others and consequently fewer signs of hormone deficiency.

MENOPAUSAL CHANGES

What physical and emotional changes occur at the menopause? The most obvious landmark of menopause is the cessation of periods. This may occur abruptly or following menstrual cycles of increasing length with decreasing menstrual flow. As ovarian hormonal function usually declines for some time before actual cessation of menses, other menopausal changes may be evident before this.

What about the woman who has had hysterectomy performed? How will she recognize menopausal changes? These symptoms fall into different groups. Women will vary in their experience of these changes because there are individual differences in both the amount of hormones that remain after menopause and the sensitivity of the body to hormonal loss.

Hot Flushes (or Flashes)

The hot flush is perhaps the most commonly experienced symptom of the menopause. About 75 per cent of women experience hot flushes after the menopause. The hot flush occurs at or soon after menopause, but in 20 per cent of women hot flushes continue for more than five years. The hot flush is generally taken to mean a feeling of warmth which passes quickly over all the body or part of it. The face, neck, and upper chest are affected most often. The feeling of warmth and 'flushing' is caused by the opening up of blood vessels in the skin. This may also produce sweating. Hot flushes may occur spontaneously or be precipitated by a warm environment, hot drinks, alcohol, and mental stress. When hot flushes are severe, a woman may awaken several times a night.

The exact cause of hot flushes is unknown. Presumably, the hormonal disturbance which occurs at the menopause produces instability of the blood vessels.

Pelvic Changes

The health of the genital organs is maintained by ovarian hormones. A lack of these hormones produces thinning of surface tissue and loss of tone of muscles. These changes may proceed over years. Both the vagina and urinary tract become more prone to infections. Symptons include itchiness, vaginal discharge, urinary frequency, and burning or discomfort on passing urine.

The thinned vagina does not lubricate with sexual arousal so that intercourse may be uncomfortable or painful.

Other Body Changes

These may not be discernible for some years after the menopause. Some women notice a gradual reduction in the size of the breasts. Backache and fractures are more common many years later as bones thin. Changes in the skin may be noticed but those caused by hormonal deficiency are perhaps less marked than the deleterious and serious effects of ageing and weather exposure.

In the past it has been unusual for women who do not smoke or take the oral contraceptive pill to have strokes or coronaries before the menopause. These disorders have occurred more frequently in males of the same age, suggesting a possible protective effect of ovarian hormones. The incidences of these cardiovascular disorders becomes similar to that of males after the menopause. Women who have experienced a premature menopause or had surgical removal of both ovaries before the age of forty and received no hormone therapy have an increased incidence of strokes and coronary disease. The situation is complex because recent studies suggest an increase in coronary disease among younger women, attributed by some to changes in women's roles with more women in the workforce and in executive positions.

Behavioural Changes

At the menopause some women experience an increase in nervousness, irritability, depression, and headaches. There may be a diminution in sexual interest, enjoyment, and orgasmic frequency. There is no increase in insanity at the menopause.

In the past there was much disagreement about whether these mood and sexual changes were a result of hormone deficiency or of the many other stresses occurring at this phase of life. It now appears that hormone deficiency at the menopause produces a state of biological vulnerability in the woman so that she may over-react to stress or even perceive events differently from before. Unfortunately, many stresses occur at this time.

STRESS IN MIDDLE AGE

During middle age, many changes occur which influence adjustment to biological changes.

Children

There may have been a stormy adolescence before children finally separate from parents and leave home. Tension points during adolescent years often centre around school progress, boyfriends or girlfriends, and morality. Conflicts may have occurred between a woman and her husband about the adolescents' behaviour. Departure of adolescents after a previously good parent/adolescent relationship may create a sense of loss in the parents. The feeling of emptiness is likely to be greater for the mother who does not have work or outside interests to fill a substantial part of her day, especially when her husband provides little satisfaction or companionship.

Recent studies suggest that the 'empty nest' syndrome is diminishing as women find satisfactory and fulfilling alternative roles.

The Marriage

After the departure of the children the couple are left to face each other alone for the first time since the first child arrived. Some couples find that their mode of communication has been through or about children. If there is little companionship or affection left, marital breakdown and divorce may result.

Alternatively, many couples value the opportunity to be alone together again without the intrusion and continued responsibility of children. A new closeness may arise with beneficial effects for husband, wife, and their relationship.

Loss

At the menopause there is a loss of fertility. Women may at this time also react to the continuing loss of youth and attractiveness. Loss of good physical health may have occurred in the parent, spouse, or close friends. Loss may lead to feelings of helplessness, hopelessness, and disappointment, especially where there have been difficulties in adapting to previous losses.

CONCLUSION

Hormonal deficiency at the menopause may lead to a number of symptoms. Hot flushes are experienced at or soon after the menopause. Pelvic symptoms may occur with the loss of health of pelvic organs. In addition, women are more biologically vulnerable to stress at this time and in our society considerable stress often occurs. Successful adjustment to these changes is necessary if women are to enjoy and use fully the remaining third of their lives. Sometimes a doctor's help is needed to help make the adjustment. Therapy often involves hormones or treatment aimed at developing coping skills or both.

The next chapter will examine the role of hormone therapy for menopausal symptoms.

9 Hormone Therapy: Effects and Side Effects

Hormone replacement therapy or HRT refers to the use of hormones at or after the menopause to compensate for the reduction in ovarian hormones which occurs at this time. Until recently HRT was almost synonymous with oestrogen therapy. Progestogens (synthetic progesterone) are now increasingly recommended. Androgens are prescribed less often.

Common questions asked are:
- Should hormones be prescribed after hysterectomy?
- What are the benefits, side effects?
- Which hormones should be prescribed?

HYSTERECTOMY AND HORMONE THERAPY

The operation of hysterectomy as such is not an indication for hormone therapy. Hormone therapy is prescribed to prevent or treat menopausal changes. Consequently, there is no need to prescribe hormones when the ovaries remain and are functioning healthily. If ovarian function is impaired, by surgical removal of the ovaries or by 'natural menopause', then administration of hormones may be considered. If the woman has already reached the menopause before hysterectomy and is not troubled by any distressing complaints, there is no need to consider hormone therapy after hysterectomy is performed.

It is necessary to weigh up the benefits and risks of hormone therapy for each woman. For many women the benefits far outweigh any side effects and for these women hormone therapy is strongly indicated. For others there are clear disadvantages to the use of a particular hormone and if troublesome symptoms occur other therapy must be considered.

BENEFITS OF HORMONE THERAPY

Relief of Symptoms

Hot flushes: Oestrogens relieve hot flushes and sweating. Progestogens also reduce the frequency and intensity of hot flushes but are not as effective as oestrogen. Some weeks of hormone therapy may be necessary before hot flushes are relieved.

Pelvic changes: Oestrogens restore the health of the vagina and lower urinary tract. Consequently, infections of these organs are hindered and the vagina lubricates more easily with sexual arousal. Intercourse becomes more comfortable. Progestogens do not have these beneficial effects on the pelvic organs.

Mood: Menopausal women taking oestrogen generally report an increased sense of well-being, feeling less irritable, tense, and depressed and better able to cope with the stresses of everyday life. Oestrogen is obviously not a panacea for mood problems which occur at the menopause. Oestrogen therapy seems to help most those women with other evidence of hormonal deficiencies (e.g. hot flushes) possibly by increasing the stability of the nervous system and making them less vulnerable to stress.

Sex: There is also growing evidence that oestrogen stimulates women's sexual interest and enjoyment. We have studied women who have had both ovaries removed at the time of hysterectomy and hence have a severe hormone deficiency. We found a beneficial effect of oestrogen on sexual interest, vaginal lubrication with arousal, sexual enjoyment, and frequency of orgasm. Progestogen had a more inhibitory effect on sexuality.

Androgens are sometimes prescribed in combination with oestrogen and seem to increase drive and enhance sexual interest and responsiveness. If sexual problems were present before the menopause, however, hormones alone are unlikely to improve the problems. Sexuality in humans is complex, and biological factors form only a part of the woman's overall response. There is more information on sexual satisfaction and how to achieve it in Chapter 3.

Skin: There is little evidence about whether oestrogen has a noticeable beneficial effect on the skin. There are different types of progestogens and some make the skin less dry or more oily.

Prevention of Complaints

Oestrogen is prescribed both for the relief of distressing symptoms and to prevent the long-term effects of hormone deficiency. The major area of prevention is that of bone loss. The effects of hormone depletion on the skeleton may not be experienced by the woman for many years. The younger the woman the more she will gain from long-term oestrogen administration. Women who experience a premature menopause or have the ovaries surgically removed before the menopause should, wherever possible, have long-term oestrogen replacement.

It is unclear whether long-term hormone therapy will prevent the adverse blood vessel changes which occur more commonly after the menopause.

DISADVANTAGES OF HORMONE THERAPY

Minor Side Effects

The most common side effects of oestrogen therapy are nausea and breast soreness and swelling. These usually respond to decreasing the amount of oestrogen taken. Nausea also improves with the duration of therapy. Acne is an unwelcome side effect of androgens and certain progestogens.

Androgens occasionally cause an increase in facial hair growth. This is more likely in those women who have a tendency to facial hair anyway. Another unwelcome but uncommon effect of androgens in the usual dose prescribed is to lower the voice.

Major Side Effects (risks)

Women with an intact uterus may bleed or menstruate when they are given hormone therapy. Such bleeding must always be investigated by the doctor to exclude the presence of disease, especially cancer. Long-term oestrogen administration may increase the risk of developing cancer of the uterus. The woman who has had her womb removed is hence at an advantage when considering hormone therapy.

Women taking long-term oestrogen therapy have the risk of developing gall-stones. A possible marginal increase in the incidence of breast cancer has been reported with long-term, high dosage oestrogen administration. It is likely that lower dosage oestrogens, cyclical administration or addition of a progestogen would decrease this risk.

Changes in the blood may lead to clot or 'thrombus' formation in women who are given hormone therapy. These clots usually lodge in veins, especially in the legs. If part of the clot detaches it can travel through blood vessels (as an embolist) and lodge somewhere where more damage can occur. Especially at risk is the brain where embolism can lead to a stroke. There have been few studies carried out to determine whether hormone replacement therapy increases the risk of thromboembolism. In younger women taking the hormones oestrogen and progestogen as the oral contraceptive pill, however, there is an increased risk of thromboembolism, especially in those who are aged over thirty-five, smoke cigarettes, and have high blood pressure. A woman who receives hormone replacement therapy usually has at least one of these risk factors, that is, age. She should do her utmost to reduce any other risk: by stopping smoking and reducing any other factors which predispose her to high blood pressure, such as obesity. Nevertheless there are differences between the oral contraceptive pill and hormone replacement therapy. In general, the woman receiving hormone replacement therapy is prescribed lower doses of hormones than those in the oral contraceptive. Wherever possible hormones are prescribed which have been shown to have the least effect on blood clotting mechanisms.

WHO SHOULD NOT RECEIVE HORMONES?

Women who have the most risk of developing side effects of oestrogen are those with a history of venous thrombosis, liver or gall-bladder disease, hyperlipidemia (high fat levels), hypertension, diabetes, personal or family history of carcinoma (cancer) of the breast or a past history of an oestrogen-dependent tumour. In any woman the presence of one or more of these risk factors must be weighed against the likely benefits of hormone therapy.

WHICH HORMONE?

Which hormones should be prescribed for a woman who has undergone hysterectomy? In general oestrogen, which has the most favourable effects in preventing long-term changes and treating distressing complaints, also carries the major risks. Where there are no contraindications, oestrogen therapy is the preferred form of hormone therapy for a woman who has had a hysterectomy. Oestrogen may be given in tablet form, as an injection, as a cream applied directly to the vagina, as a gel applied to the skin, or as a long-acting injection or implant, which may last as long as six months.

There are different types of oestrogen. The conjugated oestrogens such as conjugated equine oestrogens, oestradiol valerate and oestriol are preferable because they may have less effects on blood clotting mechanisms.

The non-conjugated oestrogens such as ethinyl oestradiol and mestranol have been used in the oral contraceptive pills and are also prescribed at the menopause.

Progestogens are recommended for two major indications. Firstly, they are prescribed for at least one week a month for the woman receiving oestrogen who still has her uterus. Progestogen used in this way helps prevent any harmful effects of oestrogen on the uterus. The woman who has had a hysterectomy will not need to take progestogen for this purpose. Secondly, a progestogen is sometimes prescribed to relieve distressing hot flushes where the use of oestrogen is contraindicated, for example, in the diabetic woman. There are many different types of progestogen available for this purpose. Progestogens may be given as tablets or as long-lasting injections. An orally active form of pure progesterone has been developed and does not have the side effects of the synthetic progestogens.

Androgens are sometimes prescribed in conjunction with oestrogen therapy. The usual indication is to help restore energy or drive and sexual interest and responsiveness. Androgen and oestrogen combinations may be given as tablets or by injection.

CLINICAL CARE WHILE TAKING HORMONES

Before you are prescribed hormones, you should have a full general examination, including having your blood pressure taken, and a breast and pelvic examination. The dosage of hormone is individually adjusted or tailored to give the minimum amount of hormone needed to relieve your symptoms. It may take one to two months for the initial relief of symptoms and an adjustment of the dose is often needed. Your doctor may tell you how to do this yourself or review your progress himself or herself.

After the dosage of hormones has been adjusted, you should visit your doctor every six months. At follow-up visits your general health and response to hormones will be assessed, and the dosage of hormones may be further adjusted. Blood pressure and breast examinations will be carried out. A pelvic examination should be carried out annually.

NON-HORMONAL DRUGS

These drugs may be prescribed for menopausal symptoms when hormone therapy is contraindicated.

Sedatives and minor tranquillizers are likely to alleviate insomnia, reduce irritability, and may reduce hot flushes, although they are not as effective as oestrogen in reducing hot flushes. Calcium, Vitamin D, and exercise may help prevent osteoporosis.

10 Life is What You Make It

Hysterectomy entails considerable psychological and physical stress. What can you do to help to adjust well to it? It is important to think what the operation means to you and to discuss your thoughts, fears, and feelings, both good and bad, with someone you can trust. Be aware that for the first six months after the operation, as your body and mind make adjustments, you may experience some fluctuation in your moods and be more easily upset than usual. This is a temporary phase and does not indicate that you are developing psychological problems. It is important to be aware that your behaviour follows your expectations of yourself. If you have negative expectations these are likely to come true, and positive expectations of the operation are likely to have beneficial effects.

DEALING WITH EMOTIONAL STRESS

Hysterectomy is only one of the stressful events you may be subjected to throughout life. Other stressful events include accidents, illnesses, bereavements, financial troubles, and problems on the job or in the family.

Here are some simple general principles for dealing with stress. Many books have been written on stress management techniques and the following points are usually highlighted. For more details you may wish to read a specific book in the further reading list.

Talk it over with someone

If something is worrying you, let it out. Talk over your worries and concerns with someone you trust: husband or close friend, father or mother, family doctor, clergyman, or psychiatrist. Talking relieves the strain and helps you bring problems into perspective. Talk to someone you feel has genuine concern for you and whom you trust.

Run away for a little while

Don't spend all your time worrying about your problems. Escape for a while into a book, television, a movie, a game. True 'escapism' can be overdone, but occasional breaks will help you see things more clearly.

Work off your anger

Give your emotions a rest by switching to physical activities. Dig up the garden. Clean out the garage. Start a hobby, join a club, go for a jog. Action is one of the best ways of dealing with tension.

Give in occasionally

If you find yourself getting into frequent quarrels, stand your ground only when you're sure you're right. Make allowances sometimes for the possibility that the other person may be right. It's easier on your body and mind to give in now and then.

Give something of yourself

Doing things for others can take your mind off your own problems. And you'll have a feeling of satisfaction and accomplishment. But do not take on impossible tasks. Find your own level.

Tackle one thing at a time

If your work load seems unbearable, do the most urgent

jobs one at a time. Put all the others aside for the time being. Learn how to take things in order.

Don't try to be always perfect

There are things you like to do best, and things that give you the most satisfaction. Give yourself a pat on the back for those you do well, but don't try to get into the Guinness Book of Records with everything you do.

Ease up on your criticism

Don't expect too much of others. Try to remember that each person has his or her own strengths, his or her own shortcomings. Trust yourself more and you will trust others.

Don't be too competitive

Often co-operation is the best approach. When you give other people a break, you often also make things easier for yourself. If they no longer feel threatened by you, they stop being a threat to you.

Make the first move

Sometimes you have the feeling that you are being left out, slighted, or rejected by others. This could be just in your imagination. If you make the first friendly move, very often others will respond. There is an old saying 'Smile and the world smiles with you, Cry and you cry alone'.

Have some fun

Too much work can be harmful. Old-fashioned play is essential for good physical and mental health. Everyone should have a sport, hobby, or outside interest that provides a complete break from the work routine.

Relaxation techniques

The technique of contracting one muscle group at a time and relaxing is a helpful one.

Tense your foot, then relax, tense your ankle, then

relax, tense your leg, then relax, tense your thigh, then relax, tense your leg, completely relax.

Tense your tummy, relax, slow your breathing, deep and even, relax, breathing slows down, deep and even, relax.

Tense your hand, relax, tense your lower arm, relax, tense your upper arm, relax, tense your shoulder, relax.

Tense your forehead muscles, relax, tense your neck muscles, relax, tense your facial muscles, relax.

Now start over again with your other leg, relax, doing the whole body again, systematically tensing and relaxing.

This exercise should only take between five and ten minutes and you should feel some benefit.

Now go through it all again, this time *only relaxing* each muscle and part of your body.

Other techniques which will help you relax include yoga, meditation, and hypnosis.

Get regular exercise

Daily exercise within your own physical limits is desirable.

Diet

A regular well-balanced diet, a little of everything, is better than a lot of one type of food. Good habits with regular meals is better than fad dieting, or starving yourself and at other times binge eating. Do not eat to comfort yourself after the operation as the weight you will gain will be no comfort. It is easy to get into bad habits of eating, for example, having coffee *and* cake with visitors. Remember that as your physical activity is somewhat reduced while you are recuperating you actually need to eat *less* not more.

DEALING WITH PHYSICAL STRESS

Some of the ways of coping with the physical stress of the operation have been dealt with in Chapter 7. These include pre-operative preparation so that you are wherever possible in good physical health before the surgery, good medical care, and allowing your body 'R & R' (rest and recuperation) leave after the operation. The following exercises may be useful to improve muscle tone before surgery and to speed physical recovery after surgery.

EXERCISES

When resting in bed, after an operation, a person may suffer from chest and leg complications if not performing regular breathing and leg exercises.

Following surgery, there may be increased mucous produced in the lungs, which may be retained when breathing is shallow and coughing difficult.

Smokers are more prone to post-operative lung congestion and infection, and are advised to stop smoking at least twenty-four hours before the operation.

Leg movements help the circulation, lessening the risk of thrombosis.

It is important that you change your position in bed from time to time to prevent continuous pressure on any one area of the body.

Foot stretching

Keeping knees straight, pull feet up and stretch feet down—ten times. See Fig. 13.

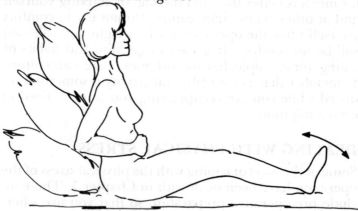

Figure 13 Position for foot stretching

Deep Breathing

With hand on lower ribs, take a deep breath in and a long slow relaxed breath out—five times.

Coughing

It is essential that sputum be removed from the chest by coughing.

Bend knees or lean forwards, support wound firmly with hands, then cough. See Fig. 14.

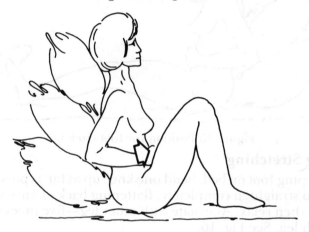

Figure 14 Position for coughing

Lying with knees bent and hands by side, raise head and shoulders then bend sideways from waist stretching right hand towards right ankle, return to starting position and relax. Repeat to the opposite side and relax. Repeat five times twice daily. Make this exercise harder by stretching to alternate sides without rest.

Continue all exercises for at least another six weeks. Exercises and activities should be performed within a pain-free range.

Make sure you have adequate daily rest.

Remember that many household jobs can be performed while sitting rather than standing (e.g. ironing, preparing vegetables).

Foot Circling

Keeping knees still, circle both feet ten times in each direction. See Fig. 15.

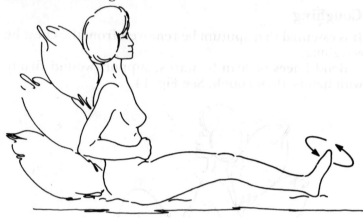

Figure 15 Position for foot circling

Leg Stretching

Keeping foot on bed, bend one knee up as far as possible, then straighten completely, flattening back of knee onto bed then relax. Alternate with other leg—five times with each leg. See Fig. 16.

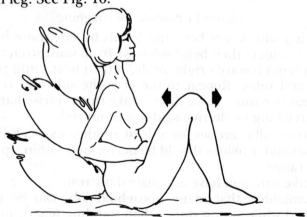

Figure 16 Position for leg stretching

Pelvic Floor Exercise

To improve the strength of the muscles which support the pelvic contents.

Lying or sitting in a comfortable position, tighten and pull up the muscles around back passage, vagina and front passage, try to hold for the count of four, then relax. Repeat five times twice a day. See Fig. 17.

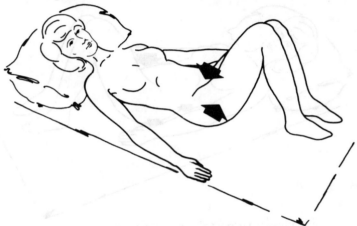

Figure 17 Position for pelvic floor exercise

Abdominal Muscle Tightening

Tighten abdominal muscles and hold for the count of four, then relax. Repeat five times twice a day.

Abdominal Muscle Strengthening

Lying with knees bent, lift head and shoulders as far as possible stretching arms towards knees and hold to the count of four then relax.

As a progression try to come up further without straining.

Stretch both arms forward across your body, aiming to touch the outside of the right knee. Hold to the count of four then relax. Repeat to outside of left knee then relax.

Repeat each exercise five times twice daily.

Pelvic Tilt Exercise

To improve posture and abdominal tone and to help relieve wind and/or backache.

Lying with knees bent, and one hand in hollow of back, tuck tail under, tighten abdominal muscles, flattening back onto hand. Hold back flat to the count of four, slowly relax. See Fig. 18.

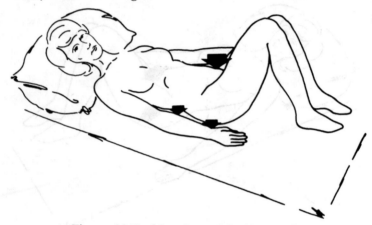

Figure 18 Position for pelvic tilt exercise

Further Reading

H. Benson, *The Relaxation Response*, Morrow, New York, 1975

A. Comfort, *The Joy of Sex: a gourmet guide to lovemaking*, Quartet, London, 1975

L. Dennerstein, G. D. Burrows, L. Cox and C. Wood, *Gynaecology, Sex and Psyche*, Melbourne University Press, Melbourne, 1978

J. Heiman, L. Lo Piccolo and J. Lo Piccolo, *Becoming Orgasmic*, Prentice Hall, New Jersey, 1976

D. Llewellyn-Jones, *Everywoman: A Gynaecological Guide for Life*, Faber, London, 1971

W. H. Utian, *The Menopause Manual: a woman's guide to the menopause*, MTP Press, Lancaster, 1978

Glossary

ADHESION Fibrous material which may form after an operation

ADRENAL Small gland above the kidney which produces a number of hormones, including sex hormones

ANALGESICS Drugs for easing moderate pain (aspirin, Panadol)

ANDROGENS Sex hormones produced in large amounts by males, in much smaller amount in all females

ANTEVERSION OF UTERUS Rotation forward

ANTICOAGULANT Drug for preventing clot formation in blood vessels

ANTI-PROSTAGLANDINS Drugs which have been found successful in preventing menstrual pain, and also prevent excessive menstrual bleeding

ARTERIOLES Tiny arteries

BEHAVIOURAL THERAPY Psychological techniques which aim to modify behaviour and often involve relaxation techniques

CANCER (non-invasive or pre-invasive) Cancer cells within the lining of the uterus but not elsewhere. 100 per cent cure possible. Treatments vary from removal of lining alone to removal of the whole uterus

CATHETER Tube passed into bladder for draining it, when there is difficulty in emptying the bladder

CERVIX The cylindrical base of the uterus, where it joins the vagina

CLOMID A drug which stimulates ovulation and reduces heavy bleeding

CLONIDINE An anti-migraine drug which reduces hot flushes

CARDIOVASCULAR DISORDER Disorder of the blood vessels or heart

COITUS Sexual intercourse

CURETTAGE A minor operation which removes the lining of the uterus

DANAZOL A drug used to reduce or stop menstruation

DEFAECATION Emptying of the bowel

DILATATION OF THE CERVIX Stretching the cervix open

DYSMENORRHOEA Severe pain during menstruation

EMBOLUS A thrombosis or other plug brought by the blood from another vessel and forced into a smaller vessel so as to obstruct circulation

EMBRYO The developing egg after fertilization

ENDOMETRIOSIS Endometrium which has spread from normal position lining the uterus to other areas in the pelvis

ENDOMETRIUM Inner lining of the uterus, which changes each month. It is shed at the time of menstruation, then grows again until pregnancy or another menstruation occurs

ETHINYL OESTRADIOL A form of oestrogen

FERTILIZATION After uniting with the sperm, the fertilized ovum forms an embryo which is held in the uterus by a mucus plug until it becomes 'implanted' in the uterus lining around the 20th day of the menstrual cycle

FETUS The developing baby before birth

FIBROIDS Lumps of muscle or fibrous material which grow within the normal muscle of the uterus, varying in size from small seeds to the size of a football. They are not a form of cancer

FIBROMYOMATA Fibroids

FISTULA An abnormal passage or communication between two internal organs or from one internal organ to the surface of the body

FOLLICLE Cyst or casing in which each egg is developed inside the ovary. Hormones (oestrogen and progesterone) are also produced by this follicle

FLUFENAMIC ACID An anti-prostaglandin

GONADOTROPHIC HORMONES Hormones which stimulate the sex glands, that is ovaries (from gonad - sex gland, trophic - nourishing)

HEPARIN A substance which prevents clotting of the blood

HORMONE A substance produced in tiny quantities in one part of the body and carried by the blood to another part where it can produce a large effect, for example, the ovaries produce oestrogen which has an effect on the uterus. Hormones are produced by glands

HORMONE REPLACEMENT THERAPY (HRT)Administration of hormones after menopause to replace those no longer produced by the ovary

HOT FLUSHES Feeling of warmth which passes quickly over the body, particularly the face, neck, and upper chest

HYPOTHALAMUS Part of the base of the brain which controls production of hormones which stimulate the ovaries and other glands

HYSTERECTOMY *Abdominal:* removal of the uterus through an incision in the abdominal wall
Extended (Wertheim's): removal of the uterus, part of the vagina and other tissues in the pelvis
Sub-total: removal of the body of the uterus but not the cervix
Total: removal of the whole uterus
Vaginal: removal of the uterus through the vagina, without an incision in the abdominal wall

LAPAROSCOPY A small operation enabling the doctor to view the pelvis through a small incision in the abdomen

LIGAMENTS Cord-like tissues partly elastic and partly muscle which hold organs in position in the cavity of the abdomen

MEFENAMIC ACID An anti-prostaglandin

MENOPAUSE, 'CHANGE OF LIFE' Cessation of menstruation

MENORRHAGIA Heavy bleeding and prolonged menstruation

MENSES Menstruation

MENSTRUAL CYCLE The period from one menstruation to the next during which hormones from the ovaries undergo regular changes

MENSTRUATION Shedding of the lining of the uterus or endometrium if pregnancy has not occurred

MESTRANOL A form of oestrogen

MICTURITION Passing of urine

MYOMECTOMY Removal of fibroids with repair of the uterus instead of removing it

NARCOTICS Pethidine, morphine or Omnopon, used as injection in cases of severe pain

OESTRADIOL VALERATE A form of oestrogen given as hormone replacement therapy

OESTRIOL A form of oestrogen given as hormone replacement therapy

OESTROGEN A hormone produced by the follicle which produces the ripening egg each month. It acts with progesterone to produce the thick lining of the uterus. Oestrogen also influences the growth and health of the genital organs, and has effects on other parts of the body

OOPHORECTOMY Removal of the ovary

ORGASM Peak of sexual excitement during the sexual act followed by profound relaxation

OSTEOPOROSIS Reduction in density of the bones, with greater fragility

OVARIAN HORMONES Oestrogen and progesterone which are produced by the particular follicle in the ovary which produces the ripe egg each month

OVARIES Organs on both sides above the uterus which produce eggs and manufacture hormones

OVULATION (time of) Time during the month when one or two ripe ova (eggs) are released from the ovaries to pass along the tube into the uterus

PERITONEUM Smooth thin material covering the outside

of the uterus

PERIPHERAL VASOCONSTRICTION Narrowing of the small arteries in the skin causing pallor and coldness in the hands and feet

PLACENTA Afterbirth

PROGESTERONE After releasing the ripe egg, this same follicle produces progesterone which together with oestrogen acts on the uterus to produce its thick lining

PROLAPSE Exaggerated dropping of the uterus when the ligaments are weakened

PROSTAGLANDINS Substances produced in the body which cause smooth muscles to contract strongly and open small blood vessels

PSYCHIATRIC ILLNESS A major disorder of the mind requiring medical care

PSYCHOLOGICAL ILLNESS Any disorder where the cause is mainly due to emotional factors such as stress

PUBERTY The time interval during which adult sex characteristics such as first menstruation appear and body growth is completed

PULMONARY Relating to the lungs

RETROVERSION OF THE UTERUS Rotation backwards

SARCOMA Cancerous like growth

SALPINGO-OOPHORECTOMY Removal of tube and ovary

SECRETION Production of substances by glands

TACHYCARDIA Rapid pulse

THROMBOEMBOLISM Blockage of a blood vessel by a blood clot which has broken loose from its site of formation

THROMBOSIS Formation of blood clot

URETER Tube carrying urine from the kidney to the bladder

UTERUS Womb

VAGINA Canal leading from the exterior of the body to the uterus

VULVA Outer area surrounding the entrance to the vagina

Index

acupuncture for menstrual pain 45
adrenal gland 102
ageing, effect on sexual activity 31-3
alcohol, effect on menstrual pain 42; effect on sexuality 33
androgens 102, 107, 109, 112
antibiotics 90
antiprostaglandins 26, 42, 48
antispasmodics for menstrual pain 45
anxiety 13, 72-4; after hysterectomy 77; and pain 45; effect on sexuality 33; treatment of 78

behaviour, hormone effects on 101
behavioural therapy for menstrual pain 45
bladder, damage to 62-3; infection of 66
bones, oestrogen effects on 100, 109
bowel, damage to 63; function after hysterectomy 66-9
breasts, hormonal effects on 100

calcium 113
cancer, of cervix 59; of ovaries 55; of uterus 54-5, 59
cardiovascular disorder 104
cervix, dilatation of 45
childbirth, effect on menstrual pain 41-2
clomiphene 48
clot (thromboembolism) 64
communication of sexual needs 31, 36-7

complications after going home 67-8
contraceptive pill 12; effect on menstrual pain 62; for excessive bleeding 47; risks for overweight patients 47; and thromboembolism 64
cost of operation 87
curettage 47; accidental damage during 55

danazol 48
danger 61-71, 85
death 70
decision for hysterectomy 56-8, 87
depression, after hysterectomy 77; effect of progestogen 47; effect on sexuality 33; and pain 45; treatment of 79, 80, 90
discharge 69, 90
doctor, choice of 90
driving 87, 90
drugs, effect on sexuality 33

embolus 64
emotions 72
emotional, adjustment 114; problems, hidden 16; response to hysterectomy 75; state and menstruation 13
endometriosis 50-2
endometrium 24, 50, 99

family, advice for 96
fears, coping with 74-5
fibroids (fibromyomata) 26, 49-50
fistula 62

flufenamic acid 48
follicle, ovarian 99

gynaecologist's decision for operation 15

hair, effect on 84
headache 41, 44
home help 87
hormone changes at menopause 101-6
hormone therapy 107; benefits of 108-9; choice of 111-12; clinical care in 112; risks of 110-11; side effects of 109
hormones, ovarian 98-101; effect of 38; see also oestrogen, progesterone
hospital, choice of 91-2
hot flushes 103, 108, 112
hypnosis for menstrual pain 45
hypochondriasis 73
hysterectomy, decision on 56-8; hazards of 61-71; preventative 17; types of 59-61

intercourse after surgery 69-70, 88

laparoscopy 45
ligaments of uterus 21
lung complications 65

masturbation 30
mefenamic acid 48
menopausal changes 102-5
menopause 97-106; hormone changes at 101-6; premature 83
menses, heavy 26
menstrual complaints, effect of alcohol and smoking on 12
menstrual cycle, effect on behaviour 101
menstrual loss, excessive 46-8
menstrual pain 40-6
menstruation 12-14, 24-6
myomectomy 50

oestrogen 23, 25, 99-102, 108-12; choice of 111; effects of 100; thrombosis risk of 47; see also ovarian hormones
oophorectomy, see removal of ovaries
operation 93
osteoporosis 113, see also bones
ovarian function, failure of 101, 102
ovarian hormones, 98-106
ovaries, cancer of 55; effect of hysterectomy on 83; infection of 54; removal of 98

pain, psychological factor in 43-5; relaxation for 45
pelvic, changes after menopause 103; infection 52
peritoneum 20
phobia, cancer 72
pituitary, gland (figure 1) 100; hormones 102
post-operative period 94-6
post-operative exercises 118-22
premature ageing 85
premenstrual tension 101
preparation, pre-operative 93
prevention of complications 71
progesterone 23, 25, 99-102; effects of 99; see also ovarian hormones
progestogen 109, 112
progestogen-only pill 47
prolapse 20
prostaglandins 23, 25
psychiatric problems 13, 76
psychological problems 13, 76

questions commonly asked 83-90

recovery after surgery 67-8
relaxation, for menstrual pain 45; techniques 116-17
response (emotional) to hysterectomy 75
risks 85

salpingo-oophorectomy 59, 98
sarcoma 50
second opinion 87
self-acceptance 35
sexual activity 26,29; effects of ageing on 31-3
sexual behaviour, hormone effects on 101
sexual desire 28
sexual drive 29
sexual knowledge 34-5
sexual intercourse, after hysterectomy 69-70, 88; frequency of 37; variety in 37
sexual response 29
sexual satisfaction, after hysterectomy 38-9; improvement in 34-5; outcome, post-operative 80-3; problems in 33
sexuality, effect of drugs and alcohol on 33
skin effect on 85, 109
smoking, effect on menstrual pain 42; and thrombosis 64-5, 111
stress, dealing with 114-18; in middle age 105; response to 76
strokes 104

thromboembolism 42
thromboembolus (clot) 64
tiredness 90

ureters, damage to 61-2
uterine muscle 22
uterus 19-24; cancer of 54-5; emotional value of 56; influence of mind on 27
vagina 20, 36; effect of oestrogen on 99; menopausal effect on 102
vitamin D 113
vulva 36, 100

wound complications 63

N H May 8 9
Ann Willios

Sally Laslet
Nursing 25
Aldwych Pub. '88

3 95

Hysterectomy